T0259135

MRI and Traumatic Brain Injury

Editors

PEJMAN JABEHDAR MARALANI
SEAN SYMONS

NEUROIMAGING CLINICS OF NORTH AMERICA

www.neuroimaging.theclinics.com

Consulting Editor
SURESH K. MUKHERJI

May 2023 • Volume 33 • Number 2

ELSEVIER

1600 John F. Kennedy Boulevard • Suite 1800 • Philadelphia, Pennsylvania, 19103-2899

http://www.neuroimaging.theclinics.com

NEUROIMAGING CLINICS OF NORTH AMERICA Volume 33, Number 2
May 2023 ISSN 1052-5149, ISBN 13: 978-0-323-97286-4

Editor: John Vassallo (j.vassallo@elsevier.com)
Developmental Editor: Karen Justine S. Dino

Neuroimaging Clinics of North America (ISSN 1052-5149) is published quarterly by Elsevier Inc., 360 Park Avenue South, New York, NY 10010-1710. Months of issue are February, May, August, and November. Business and editorial offices: 1600 John F. Kennedy Blvd., Suite 1800, Philadelphia, PA 19103-2899. Business and editorial offices: 6277 Sea Harbor Drive, Orlando, FL 32887-4800. Periodicals postage paid at New York, NY, and additional mailing offices. Subscription prices are USD 413 per year for US individuals, USD 745 per year for US institutions, USD 100 per year for US students and residents, USD 483 per year for Canadian individuals, USD 949 per year for Canadian institutions, USD 562 per year for international individuals, USD 949 per year for international institutions, USD 100 per year for Canadian students and residents and USD 260 per year for foreign students and residents. To receive student/resident rate, orders must be accompanied by name of affiliated institution, date of term, and the *signature* of program/residency coordinator on institution letterhead. Orders will be billed at individual rate until proof of status is received. Foreign air speed delivery is included in all *Clinics* subscription prices. All prices are subject to change without notice. POSTMASTER: Send address changes to *Neuroimaging Clinics of North America*, Elsevier Health Sciences Division, Subscription **Customer Service, 3251 Riverport Lane, Maryland Heights, MO 63043. Telephone: 1-800-654-2452 (U.S. and Canada); 314-447-8871 (outside U.S. and Canada). Fax: 314-447-8029. E-mail: journalscustomerservice-usa@elsevier.com (for print support); journals onlinesupport-usa@elsevier.com (for online support).**

Reprints. For copies of 100 or more of articles in this publication, please contact the Commercial Reprints Department, Elsevier Inc., 360 Park Avenue South, New York, NY 10010-1710. Tel.: 212-633-3874; Fax: 212-633-3820; E-mail: reprints@elsevier.com.

Neuroimaging Clinics of North America is covered by *Excerpta Medical/EMBASE,* the RSNA Index of Imaging Literature, *MEDLINE/PubMed (Index Medicus),* MEDLINE/MEDLARS, SciSearch, Research Alert, and Neuroscience Citation Index.

PROGRAM OBJECTIVE

The goal of *Neuroimaging Clinics of North America* is to keep practicing radiologists and radiology residents up to date with current clinical practice in radiology by providing timely articles reviewing the state of the art in patient care.

TARGET AUDIENCE

Practicing radiologists, radiology residents, and other healthcare professionals who utilize neuroimaging findings to provide patient care.

LEARNING OBJECTIVES

Upon completion of this activity, participants will be able to:
1. Review clinical updates in traumatic brain injury and head trauma in children and adults.
2. Discuss conventional MRI imaging and other imaging approaches for the management of traumatic brain injuries.
3. Recognize abusive head trauma in children with imaging studies.

ACCREDITATION

The Elsevier Office of Continuing Medical Education (EOCME) is accredited by the Accreditation Council for Continuing Medical Education (ACCME) to provide continuing medical education for physicians.

The EOCME designates this journal-based CME activity for a maximum of 11 *AMA PRA Category 1 Credit*(s)™. Physicians should claim only the credit commensurate with the extent of their participation in the activity.

All other healthcare professionals requesting continuing education credit for this enduring material will be issued a certificate of participation.

DISCLOSURE OF CONFLICTS OF INTEREST

The EOCME assesses conflict of interest with its instructors, faculty, planners, and other individuals who are in a position to control the content of CME activities. All relevant conflicts of interest that are identified are thoroughly vetted by EOCME for fair balance, scientific objectivity, and patient care recommendations. EOCME is committed to providing its learners with CME activities that promote improvements or quality in healthcare and not a specific proprietary business or a commercial interest.

The planning committee, staff, authors, and editors listed below have identified no financial relationships or relationships to products or devices they or their spouse/life partner have with commercial interest related to the content of this CME activity:

Mohit Agarwal, MD, DABR; Ibrahem Albalkhi; Ulas Bagci, PhD; Asthik Biswas, MBBS, DNB; Helen Branson, BSc, MBBS, FRANZCR; Nathan W. Churchill, PhD; Ange Diouf, MD, FRCPC; David Douglas, MD; Simon J. Graham, PhD; Matthew Grant, MD; E. Mark Haacke, PhD; Charlie Chia-Tsong Hsu, MBBS, FRANZCR; Lynette Jones, MSN, RN-BC; Anish Kapadia, MD; Venkatagiri Krishnamurthy, PhD; Pradeep Krishnan, MBBS, MD; Pradeep Kuttysankaran; Michael H. Lev, MD, FAHA, FACR; JiaJing Liu, MD, PhD; Matylda Machnowska, MD, FRCPC; Mary D. Maher, MD; Kshitij Mankad, MBBS, FRCR; Pejman Jabehdar Maralani, MD, FRCPC; Claudia Martinez-Rios, MD; David Mikulis, MD; Saeedeh Mirbagheri, MD; Suyash Mohan, MD, PDCC; Megan Moore, CRNP; Daniel Ryan, MD; Danielle K. Sandsmark, MD, PhD; Tom A. Schweizer, PhD; Sean K. Sethi, MS; Manohar Shroff, MD, FRCPC, DABR, DMRD; Sean P. Symons, MD; Madhura Tamhankar, MD; Jeffrey B. Ware, MD; Max Wintermark, MD; Erin T. Wong, MD; Noushin Yahyavi-Firouz-Abadi, MD

UNAPPROVED/OFF-LABEL USE DISCLOSURE

The EOCME requires CME faculty to disclose to the participants:
1. When products or procedures being discussed are off-label, unlabelled, experimental, and/or investigational (not US Food and Drug Administration [FDA] approved), and
2. Any limitations on the information presented, such as data that are preliminary or that represent ongoing research, interim analyses, and/or unsupported opinions. Faculty may discuss information about pharmaceutical agents that is outside of FDA-approved labelling. This information is intended solely for CME and is not intended to promote off-label use of these medications. If you have any questions, contact the medical affairs department of the manufacturer for the most recent prescribing information.

TO ENROLL

To enroll in the *Neuroimaging Clinics of North America* Continuing Medical Education program, call customer service at 1-800-654-2452 or sign up online at http://www.theclinics.com/home/cme. The CME program is available to subscribers for an additional annual fee of USD 254.00.

METHOD OF PARTICIPATION

In order to claim credit, participants must complete the following:
1. Complete enrolment as indicated above.
2. Read the activity.

3. Complete the CME Test and Evaluation. Participants must achieve a score of 70% on the test. All CME Tests and Evaluations must be completed online.

CME INQUIRIES/SPECIAL NEEDS

For all CME inquiries or special needs, please contact elsevierCME@elsevier.com.

NEUROIMAGING CLINICS OF NORTH AMERICA

THE CLINICS ARE AVAILABLE ONLINE!
Access your subscription at:
www.theclinics.com

Contributors

CONSULTING EDITOR

SURESH K. MUKHERJI, MD, MBA, FACR
Clinical Professor, Marian University, Director of Head and Neck Radiology, ProScan Imaging, Regional Medical Director, Envision Physician Services, Carmel, Indiana, USA

EDITORS

PEJMAN JABEHDAR MARALANI, MD
Associate Professor of Radiology, Division of Neuroradiology, Department of Medical Imaging, University of Toronto, Sunnybrook Health Sciences Centre, Toronto, Ontario, Canada

SEAN SYMONS, MD, MPH
Associate Professor of Radiology, Division of Neuroradiology, Department of Medical Imaging, University of Toronto, Sunnybrook Health Sciences Centre, Toronto, Ontario, Canada

AUTHORS

MOHIT AGARWAL, MD
Assistant Professor of Radiology, Division of Neuroradiology, Department of Radiology, Medical College of Wisconsin, Milwaukee, Wisconsin, USA

IBRAHEM ALBALKHI
Department of Neuroradiology, Great Ormond Street Hospital for Children NHS Foundation Trust, London, United Kingdom; College of Medicine, Alfaisal University, Riyadh, Kingdom of Saudi Arabia

ULAS BAGCI, PhD
Radiology and Biomedical Engineering Department, Northwestern University, Chicago, Illinois, USA; Department of Computer Science, University of Central Florida

ASTHIK BISWAS, MBBS, DNB
Department of Diagnostic Imaging, The Hospital for Sick Children, Department of Medical Imaging, University of Toronto, Ontario, Canada; Neuroradiologist, Department of Neuroradiology, Great Ormond Street Hospital for Children NHS Foundation Trust, London, United Kingdom

HELEN M. BRANSON, BSc, MBBS, FRANZCR
Pediatric Neuroradiologist, Department of Diagnostic Imaging, SickKids, Assistant Professor, University of Toronto, Toronto, Ontario, Canada

NATHAN W. CHURCHILL, PhD
Neuroscience Research Program, Saint Michael's Hospital, Keenan Research Centre for Biomedical Science of Saint Michael's Hospital, Physics Department, Toronto Metropolitan University, Toronto, Ontario, USA

ANGE DIOUF, MD, FRCPC
Master's Degree Candidate in Biomedical Sciences, University of Montreal, Department of Radiology, Centre Hospitalier de l'Universite de Montreal (CHUM), Montreal, Quebec, Canada; Interventional Neuroradiology Clinical Fellow at St. Michael's Hospital, University of Toronto, Toronto, Ontario, Canada

DAVID DOUGLAS, MD
Department of Radiology, Stanford University, Palo Alto, California, USA; Department of Radiology, 96th Medical Group, Eglin Air Force Base

SIMON J. GRAHAM, PhD
Department of Medical Biophysics, University of Toronto, Hurvitz Brain Sciences Program, Sunnybrook Research Institute, Physical Sciences Platform, Sunnybrook Research Institute, Toronto, Ontario, USA

MATTHEW GRANT, MD
Department of Radiology, Stanford University, Palo Alto, California, USA; Department of Radiology, Uniformed Services University of the Health Sciences, Department of Radiology, Landstuhl Regional Medical Center

E. MARK HAACKE, PhD
Departments of Radiology and Neurology, Wayne State University School of Medicine

CHARLIE CHIA-TSONG HSU, MBBS, FRANZCR
Division of Neuroradiology, Department of Medical Imaging, Gold Coast University Hospital, Australia; Division of Neuroradiology, Lumus Imaging, Varsity Lakes Day Hospital, Gold Coast, Australia

ANISH KAPADIA, MD
Department of Medical Imaging, University of Toronto, Department of Medical Imaging, Sunnybrook Health Sciences Centre, Toronto, Ontario, Canada

VENKATAGIRI KRISHNAMURTHY, PhD
Department of Medicine, Division of Geriatrics and Gerontology, Department of Neurology, Emory University, Atlanta, Georgia, USA; Center for Visual and Neurocognitive Rehabilitation, Atlanta Veterans Affairs Medical Center (VAMC), Decatur, Georgia, USA

PRADEEP KRISHNAN, MBBS, MD
Neuroradiologist, Department of Diagnostic Imaging, The Hospital for Sick Children, Assistant Professor, Department of Medical Imaging, University of Toronto, Ontario, Canada

MICHAEL H. LEV, MD, FAHA, FACR
Director Emergency Radiology, Massachusetts General Hospital, Professor of Radiology, Harvard Medical School, Boston, Massachusetts, USA

JIAJING LIU, MD, PhD
Department of Radiology, Stanford University, Palo Alto, California, USA

MATYLDA MACHNOWSKA, MD, FRCPC
Assistant Professor, Diagnostic Neuroradiology Program Director, Department of Medical Imaging, University of Toronto, Toronto, Ontario, Canada

MARY D. MAHER, MD
Assistant Professor of Radiology, Division of Neuroradiology, Department of Radiology, Perelman School of Medicine, University of Pennsylvania, Philadelphia, Pennsylvania, USA

KSHITIJ MANKAD, MBBS, FRCR
Neuroradiologist, Department of Neuroradiology, Great Ormond Street Hospital for Children NHS Foundation Trust, London, United Kingdom; Associate Professor, UCL GOS Institute of Child Health

CLAUDIA MARTINEZ-RIOS, MD
Pediatric Radiologist, Department of Diagnostic Imaging, SickKids, Assistant Professor, University of Toronto, Toronto, Ontario, Canada; Pediatric Neuroradiologist, Department of Medical Imaging, CHEO, Assistant Professor, University of Ottawa, Ottawa, Ontario, Canada

DAVID J. MIKULIS, MD
Professor and Director of the JDMI Functional Cerebrovascular Research Lab, Senior Scientist Krembil Research Institute, Department of Medical Imaging, University of Toronto, The University Health Network and The Toronto Western Hospital, Toronto, Ontario, Canada

SAEEDEH MIRBAGHERI, MD
Assistant Professor of Radiology, University of Vermont Medical Center, Burlington, Vermont, USA

SUYASH MOHAN, MD, PDCC
Associate Professor of Radiology, Associate Professor of Neurosurgery, Division of Neuroradiology, Departments of Radiology and Neurosurgery, Perelman School of Medicine, University of Pennsylvania, Philadelphia, Pennsylvania, USA

MEGAN MOORE, CRNP
Department of Neurology, Perelman School of Medicine, University of Pennsylvania, Philadelphia, Pennsylvania, USA

DANIEL RYAN, MD
Adjunct Assistant Professor of Radiology,
Southern Illinois University School of Medicine,
Springfield, Illinois, USA

DANIELLE K. SANDSMARK, MD, PhD
Assistant Professor, Department of Neurology,
Division of Neurocritical Care, Perelman
School of Medicine, University of
Pennsylvania, Philadelphia, Pennsylvania, USA

TOM A. SCHWEIZER, PhD
Neuroscience Research Program, Saint
Michael's Hospital, Keenan Research Centre
for Biomedical Science of Saint Michael's
Hospital, Faculty of Medicine (Neurosurgery),
University of Toronto, Toronto, Ontario, USA

SEAN K. SETHI, MS
Department of Radiology, Wayne State
University School of Medicine

**MANOHAR SHROFF, MD, FRCPC, DABR,
DMRD**
Neuroradiologist, Department of Diagnostic
Imaging, The Hospital for Sick Children,
Professor, Department of Medical Imaging,
University of Toronto, Ontario, Canada

MADHURA A. TAMHANKAR, MD
Associate Professor of Ophthalmology,
Division of Neuro-Ophthalmology, Department
of Ophthalmology, Perelman School of
Medicine, University of Pennsylvania,
Philadelphia, Pennsylvania, USA

JEFFREY B. WARE, MD
Assistant Professor, Department of Radiology,
Neuroradiology Division, University of
Pennsylvania, Philadelphia, Pennsylvania, USA

MAX WINTERMARK, MD
Department of Radiology, Stanford University,
Palo Alto, California, USA; Neuroradiology
Department, The University of Texas MD
Anderson Cancer Center, Houston, Texas,
USA

ERIN T. WONG, MD
Department of Medical Imaging, University of
Toronto, Department of Medical Imaging,
Sunnybrook Health Sciences Centre, Toronto,
Ontario, Canada

NOUSHIN YAHYAVI-FIROUZ-ABADI, MD
Associate Professor of Radiology and Nuclear
Medicine, University of Maryland School of
Medicine, Baltimore, Maryland, USA

Contents

MR imaging has been shown to have higher sensitivity than computed tomography (CT) for traumatic intracranial soft tissue injuries as well as most cases of intracranial hemorrhage, thus making it a significant adjunct to CT in the management of traumatic brain injury, mostly in the subacute to chronic phase, but may also be of use in the acute phase, when there are persistent neurologic symptoms unexplained by prior imaging.

Traumatic brain injury (TBI) is a major cause of death and disability in children across the world. The aim of initial brain trauma management of pediatric patients is to diagnose the extent of TBI and to determine if immediate neurosurgical intervention is required. A noncontrast computed tomography is the recommended diagnostic imaging choice for all patients with acute moderate to severe TBI. This article outlines the current use of conventional MR imaging in the management of pediatric head trauma and discusses potential future recommendations.

The acute and long-term neurobiological sequelae of concussion (mild traumatic brain injury [mTBI]) and sub-concussive head trauma have become increasingly apparent in recent decades in part due to neuroimaging research. Although imaging has an established role in the clinical management of mTBI for the identification of intracranial lesions warranting urgent interventions, MR imaging is increasingly employed for the detection of post-traumatic sequelae which carry important prognostic significance. As neuroimaging research continues to elucidate the pathophysiology of TBI underlying prolonged recovery and the development of persistent post-concussive symptoms, there is a strong motivation to translate these techniques into clinical use for improved diagnosis and therapeutic monitoring.

Traumatic brain injury (TBI) affects > 3 million people in the United States annually. Although the number of deaths related to severe TBIs has stabalized, mild TBIs, often termed concussions, are increasing. As evidence indicates that a significant proportion of these mild injuries are associated with long-lasting functional deficits that impact work performance, social integration, and may predispose to later cognitive decline, it is important that we (a) recognize these injuries, (b) identify those at highest risk of poor recovery, and (c) initiate appropriate treatments promptly. We discuss the epidemiology of TBI, the most common persistent symptoms, and treatment approaches.

Advanced imaging techniques are needed to assist in providing a prognosis for patients with traumatic brain injury (TBI), particularly mild TBI (mTBI). Diffusion tensor imaging (DTI) is one promising advanced imaging technique, but has shown variable results in patients with TBI and is not without limitations, especially when considering individual patients. Efforts to resolve these limitations are being explored and include developing advanced diffusion techniques, creating a normative database, improving study design, and testing machine learning algorithms. This article will review the fundamentals of DTI, providing an overview of the current state of its utility in evaluating and providing prognosis in patients with TBI.

In this review, we discuss the basics of functional MRI (fMRI) techniques including task-based and resting state fMRI, and overview the major findings in patients with traumatic brain injury. We summarize the studies that have longitudinally evaluated the changes in brain connectivity and task-related activation in trauma patients during different phases of trauma. We discuss how these data may potentially be used for prognostication, treatment planning, or monitoring and management of trauma patients.

The mechanisms for regulating cerebral blood flow (CBF) are highly sensitive to traumatic brain injury (TBI). Perfusion imaging techniques technique may be used to assess CBF and identify perfusion abnormalities following a TBI. Studies have identified CBF disturbances across the injury severity spectrum and correlations with both acute and long-term indices of clinical outcome. Although not yet widely used in the clinical context, this is an important area of ongoing research.

Mary D. Maher, Mohit Agarwal, Madhura A. Tamhankar, and Suyash Mohan

Traumatic brain injury disrupts the complex anatomy of the afferent and efferent visual pathways. Injury to the afferent pathway can result in vision loss, visual field deficits, and photophobia. Injury to the efferent pathway primarily causes eye movement abnormalities resulting in ocular misalignment and double vision. Injury to both the afferent and efferent systems can result in significant visual disability.

Erin T. Wong, Anish Kapadia, Venkatagiri Krishnamurthy, and David J. Mikulis

Cerebrovascular reactivity (CVR) reflects the change in cerebral blood flow in response to vasodilatory stimuli enabling assessment of the health of the cerebral vasculature. Recent advances in the quantitative delivery of CO_2 stimuli with computer-controlled sequential gas delivery have enabled mapping of the speed and magnitude of response to flow stimuli. These CVR advances when applied to patients with acute concussion have unexpectedly shown faster speed and greater magnitude of responses unseen in other diseases that typically show the opposite effects. The strength of the CVR alterations have diagnostic potential in single subjects with AUC values in the 0.90-0.94 range.

Charlie Chia-Tsong Hsu, Sean K. Sethi, and E. Mark Haacke

Susceptibility-weighted imaging (SWI) is a MR imaging technique suited to detect structural and microstructural abnormalities in traumatic brain injury (TBI). This review article provide an insight in to the physics principles of SWI and its clinical application in unraveling the complex interaction of the biophysical mechanisms of head injury. Literature evidences support SWI as the most ideal sequence in detection of microbleeds, which is the "tip of the iceberg" biomarker of microvascular injuries. The review also detailed the emerging advance techniques of Quantitative susceptibility mapping (QSM) and artificial intelligence offer the ability to detect and follow the evolution of microbleeds in patient with chronic TBI. These new techniques offers a unique insight into the acute and chronic state of TBI.

Asthik Biswas, Pradeep Krishnan, Ibrahem Albalkhi, Kshitij Mankad, and Manohar Shroff

In this article, we describe relevant anatomy, mechanisms of injury, and imaging findings of abusive head trauma (AHT). We also briefly address certain mimics of AHT, controversies, pearls, and pitfalls. Concepts of injury, its evolution, and complex nature of certain cases are highlighted with the help of case vignettes.

Foreword
MRI and Traumatic Brain Injury

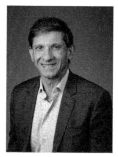

Suresh K. Mukherji, MD, MBA, FACR
Consulting Editor

Drs Pejman Maralani and Sean Symons eloquently and accurately describe in their Preface the substantial socioeconomic impact of traumatic brain injury (TBI). Our understanding of the biologic basis of TBI is evolving, and the initial diagnostic modalities, such as computed tomography, have been augmented by techniques that measure functional and metabolic alterations resulting from the traumatic injury. The individual and socioeconomic sequelae of TBI have also raised concerns about the involvement of the medicolegal community and the need to ensure we have proper health care resources to improve TBI prognosis.

It is with this in mind that we decided to devote an issue of *Neuroimaging Clinics* to TBI with a specific emphasis on MR imaging. There are articles covering the diagnostic utility of standard and advanced MR imaging techniques in TBI, which include diffusion tensor imaging, functional MR imaging, perfusion MR imaging, cerebrovascular reactivity, and susceptibility weighted imaging/quantitative susceptibility

mapping, and an article focused on pediatric brain trauma. This issue also has an article describing the clinical impact of concussion and an article looking into the future of TBI imaging.

I would especially like to thank Drs Maralani and Symons for being Guest Editors and creating this important issue. TBI is a very complex topic with many "layers," and they have done a fantastic job identifying and organizing the most important topics. The articles are amazing, and I would like to thank all of the article authors for their wonderful contributions. This is a unique topic, and I thank Drs Maralani and Symons and all the article authors for this very special issue.

Suresh K. Mukherji, MD, MBA, FACR
Marian University, Head and Neck Radiology
ProScan Imaging, Carmel, IN 46032, USA

E-mail address:
sureshmukherji@hotmail.com

Neuroimag Clin N Am 33 (2023) xv
https://doi.org/10.1016/j.nic.2023.02.001
1052-5149/23/© 2023 Published by Elsevier Inc.

Preface

MRI and Traumatic Brain Injury

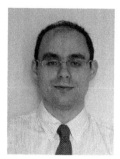 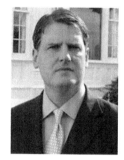

Pejman Jabehdar Maralani, MD   Sean Symons, MD, MPH

Editors

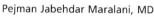

Traumatic brain injury (TBI) occurs when an injury disrupts the normal function of the brain.[1] There were more than 233,000 hospitalizations in 2019 and 64,000 deaths in 2020 in the United States as a result of TBI.[2] Globally, TBI is estimated to cost $400 billion annually.[3] TBI incurs major health care costs in both acute, subacute, and chronic stages. In addition to direct and indirect costs of medical care related to long-term complications, TBI has major socioeconomic impacts in terms of lost productivity and quality of life.

Our understanding of pathophysiology of TBI has significantly changed in recent years. While the effect of mechanical forces and acute hemorrhages in different intracranial compartments, associated mass effects, and their consequences are the main areas of concern in acute care, secondary injury mechanisms from oxidative stress, excitotoxic damage, and neuroinflammation are now known to play a role in acute and long-term pathophysiology of TBI.[4]

With regards to imaging, in acute TBI, computed tomographic (CT) scan is still the modality of choice due to widespread access, short image acquisition times, and its ability to demonstrate major intracranial findings that need urgent surgical interventions. MR imaging in the acute stage is primarily reserved when the clinical findings cannot be explained by the findings from CT scan. However, with advances in MR imaging technology, the

imaging acquisition times are getting shorter, increasing feasibility of MR imaging use in the acute setting as demonstrated by the growing number of MR imaging scanners in North American hospitals. However, there is a very large body of literature on the use of MR imaging in subacute and chronic stages of TBI for prognostication and prediction of long-term outcome. Advanced MR imaging techniques, such as diffusion tensor imaging (DTI), functional MR imaging (fMR imaging), perfusion MR imaging, cerebrovascular reactivity (CVR), and susceptibility weighted imaging/quantitative susceptibility mapping (SWI/qSM), have been extensively studied to assess microstructural integrity/damage and neurovascular coupling and metabolic changes of the brain. While the results are very promising, there is large heterogeneity in the conduct of these studies. Consistent and uniform study designs and imaging protocols can unravel more mysteries in future studies.

This issue of *Neuroimaging Clinics* provides a comprehensive review of the use of MR imaging in acute and nonacute TBI. Initially, the role of conventional MR imaging in TBI in adults and children is reviewed followed by articles on imaging approach to TBI and clinical updates on concussion. This is complemented by the review of advanced MR imaging applications in TBI, including DTI, fMR imaging, perfusion MR imaging, CVR, and SWI/qSM. The collection also has two unique articles

Neuroimag Clin N Am 33 (2023) xvii–xviii
https://doi.org/10.1016/j.nic.2023.01.012
1052-5149/23/© 2023 Published by Elsevier Inc.

on TBI and vision and on imaging of nonaccidental injury in children, further highlighting the role of MR imaging in TBI.

We would like to sincerely thank the authors for their dedication and for sharing their expertise in this issue of *Neuroimaging Clinics*.

Pejman Jabehdar Maralani, MD
Division of Neuroradiology
Department of Medical Imaging
University of Toronto
Sunnybrook Health Sciences Centre
AG270C-2075 Bayview Avenue
Toronto, ON M4N 3M5, Canada

Sean Symons, MD, MPH
Division of Neuroradiology
Department of Medical Imaging
University of Toronto
Sunnybrook Health Sciences Centre
MG167-2075 Bayview Avenue
Toronto, ON M4N 3M5, Canada

E-mail addresses:
pejman.maralani@sunnybrook.ca (P.J. Maralani)
sean.symons@sunnybrook.ca (S. Symons)

REFERENCES

1. Marr AL, Coronado VG. Central nervous system injury surveillance data submission standards—2002. Atlanta (GA): US Department of Health and Human Services, CDC; 2004.
2. Centers for Disease Control and Prevention, National Center for Injury Prevention and Control. Traumatic brain injury & concussion. Available at: https://www.cdc.gov/traumaticbraininjury/data/index.html. Accessed October 31, 2022.
3. Maas AIR, Menon DK, Adelson PD, et al. Traumatic brain injury: integrated approaches to improve prevention, clinical care, and research. Lancet Neurol 2017;16(12):987–1048. https://doi.org/10.1016/S1474-4422(17)30371-X.
4. Atkins EJ, Newman NJ, Biousse V. Post-traumatic visual loss. Rev Neurol Dis 2008;5(2):73–81.

Introduction

MRI and Traumatic Brain Injury: Where Are We Heading?

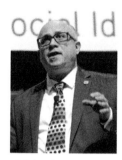

Michael H. Lev, MD

Traumatic brain injury (TBI) is currently very much in the public consciousness. A quick Google search reveals over 150 million TBI-related hits, including several National Institute of Neurological Disorders and Stroke, Department of Defense, and even National Football League (NFL) funded initiatives, such as the National Institutes of Health–sponsored TRACK-TBI study. I was therefore delighted when Drs Maralani and Symons invited me to write this introduction for their issue on "MRI and Traumatic Brain Injury," for this issue of the *Neuroimaging Clinics* series.

Indeed, in response to headlines, such as "*ninety-nine percent of ailing NFL player brains show hallmarks of neurodegenerative disease, autopsy study finds*" (from a 2017 *JAMA* study),[1] NFL efforts this past summer have called for modified helmet and other training policies aimed at reducing the rate of head injuries. The 2022 updated Official Playing Rules, for example, specify (i) declaring a penalty "*if a player lowers his head and makes forcible contact with his helmet against an opponent,*" and (ii) requiring all linemen, tight ends, and linebackers to wear padded "Guardian Caps" outside their helmets during training, which can reduce the severity of head impacts by at least 20% when worn by both players during a collision.[2] Most recently, in early October 2022, the NFL and NFL Players Association further updated their protocols, to prohibit players with ataxia from reentering games following concussive injury (perhaps in part addressing the query posed in the title of this introduction, "*where are we heading*?"; pun intended).[3]

Moreover, chronic traumatic encephalopathy (CTE), first reported back in 2009, is an additional evolving topic, considered in the context of sports injury, for which imaging is likely to play an increasing role.[4,5] In this regard, readers are encouraged to watch the two-part, 2013 Frontline episode titled, "*League of Denial: The NFL's Concussion Crisis,*"[6] which aired almost 9 years to the day before this past week's NFL rule changes. Premortem diagnosis of CTE is likely to feature Tau-PET imaging, which strongly correlates with postmortem, histologically confirmed, CTE-related tau neuropathology.[7–9]

This issue of *Neuroimaging Clinics* focuses on advanced imaging for diagnosis and prognosis, with articles covering conventional MR imaging in adults and children, diffusion-weighted imaging and diffusion-tensor imaging, functional MR imaging, perfusion MR imaging, cerebrovascular reactivity and susceptibility-weighted imaging with quantitative susceptibility mapping, as well as more clinically focused articles including pediatric nonaccidental trauma.

Finally, despite this focus on TBI diagnosis/prognosis using advanced imaging and, more recently, serum biomarkers, rather than treatment, it is

Neuroimag Clin N Am 33 (2023) xix–xx
https://doi.org/10.1016/j.nic.2022.12.002
1052-5149/23/© 2022 Published by Elsevier Inc.

noteworthy that imaging has provided pilot clinical trial data supporting a potential therapy for patients with moderate TBI.[10] Specifically, preliminary studies have suggested that "transcranial near-infrared low-level light therapy (LLLT) administered after traumatic brain injury (TBI) confers a neuroprotective response," possibly mediated through a myelin repair pathway mechanism. Figueiro Longo and colleagues, in a randomized, prospective, double-blind, placebo-controlled, single-center trial of 68 patients with moderate TBI (2015–2019), administered LLLT within 72 hours of traumatic injury and performed serial MR imaging at acute (<72 hours), early subacute (2–3 weeks), and late subacute (~3 months) time points. In the 28 patients randomized to LLLT (vs sham) who completed at least one treatment session, LLLT statistically significantly altered multiple diffusion-tensor imaging parameters in the late subacute stage, providing evidence that light therapy may impact physiologic mechanisms involved in neuronal repair, and that diffusion MR imaging may provide a biomarker for following treatment response.

In conclusion, TBI is a major global public health issue, with annual incidence estimated to be 27 to 69 million individuals, many with substantial disabilities, resulting in significant socioeconomic costs worldwide.[11] Drs Maralani and Symons' issue on "MRI and Traumatic Brain Injury" provides timely, cutting-edge reviews and updates on advanced imaging of TBI, and as such, is a welcome addition to the literature on this topic. They and their authors are to be congratulated!

Michael H. Lev, MD, FAHA, FACR

Massachusetts General Hospital, Harvard Medical School, 55 Fruit Street, Boston, MA 02114, USA

E-mail address:
mlev@partners.org

REFERENCES

1. Mez J, Daneshvar DH, Kiernan PT, et al. Clinicopathological evaluation of chronic traumatic encephalopathy in players of American football. JAMA 2017; 318(4):360–70.

2. Fortier S. and Maske M., These puffy helmet caps are the next big thing in NFL player safety, Available at: https://www.washingtonpost.com/sports/2022/08/19/nfl-guardian-caps-concussions/. Accessed January 16, 2023.

3. Maske M., NFL, NFLPA change concussion protocols, complete Tua Tagovailoa review, Available at: https://www.washingtonpost.com/sports/2022/10/08/tua-tagovailoa-nfl-investigation-protocols/. Accessed January 16, 2023.

4. McKee AC, Cantu RC, Nowinski CJ, et al. Chronic traumatic encephalopathy in athletes: progressive tauopathy after repetitive head injury. J Neuropathol Exp Neurol 2009;68(7): 709–35.

5. Omalu BI, Bailes J, Hammers JL, et al. Chronic traumatic encephalopathy, suicides and parasuicides in professional American athletes: the role of the forensic pathologist. Am J Forensic Med Pathol 2010;31(2):130–2.

6. Alosco ML, Su Y, Stein TD, et al, Diagnose C. T. E. Research Project. Associations between near end-of-life flortaucipir PET and postmortem CTE-related tau neuropathology in six former American football players. Eur J Nucl Med Mol Imaging 2022. Epub ahead of print.

7. Kirk M., Gilmore J., Wiser M., FRONTLINE PBS television program titled, LEAGUE OF DENIAL: THE NFL'S CONCUSSION CRISIS, https://www.pbs.org/wgbh/frontline/documentary/league-of-denial/. Accessed January 16, 2023.

8. Mantyh WG, Spina S, Lee A, et al. Tau positron emission tomographic findings in a former US football player with pathologically confirmed chronic traumatic encephalopathy. JAMA Neurol 2020;77(4): 517–21.

9. Stern RA, Adler CH, Chen K, et al. Tau positron-emission tomography in former National Football League players. N Engl J Med 2019;380(18): 1716–25.

10. Figueiro Longo MG, Tan CO, Chan S-T, et al. Effect of transcranial low-level light therapy vs sham therapy among patients with moderate traumatic brain injury: a randomized clinical trial. JAMA Netw Open 2020;3(9):e2017337.

11. Dewan MC, Rattani A, Gupta S, et al. Estimating the global incidence of traumatic brain injury. J Neurosurg 2018;1–18.

Conventional MR Imaging in Trauma Management in Adults

Ange Diouf, MD, FRCPC[a,b,c], Matylda Machnowska, MD, FRCPC[d,*]

KEYWORDS

- MR imaging • Computed tomography (CT) • Trauma • Management • Adult • Contusion
- Diffuse axonal injury (DAI)

KEY POINTS

- Brain MR imaging is an important adjunct to CT in the context of trauma, especially regarding early detection of focal intra-axial primary or secondary injuries, such as diffuse axonal injury, edema, infarction, or fat emboli, which can have little to no correlation on CT in the acute phase.
- Although most extra-axial injuries are readily detectable on CT, MR imaging shows similar versus slightly higher sensitivity for some extra-axial hemorrhages, especially in the subacute and chronic phases.
- Recent advances in image acquisition strategy have supported the rapidly increased use of MR imaging in trauma patients.

INTRODUCTION

Over 2 million Americans are evaluated in the emergency room every year for traumatic brain injury (TBI),[1,2] which results in upward of 250,000 hospitalizations and 50,000 TBI-related deaths in the United States every year[3]. Most of these emergency visits and hospitalizations in 2013 were related to falls, whereas the majority of deaths were related to self-harm, with motor vehicle accidents as a close second.[2]

Although CT remains the initial modality of choice for detecting acute lesions requiring urgent treatment in the context of TBI (given ease of access, lower imaging cost, faster imaging time, and better evaluation of bony anatomy), MR imaging represents an important adjunct in diagnosing nonsurgical lesions in medically stable patients, in order to better guide medical management and predict degree of neurologic recovery,[4,5] as evidenced by the ever increasing use of MR imaging in North

American emergency departments.[6] In fact, MR imaging in the context of TBI is not only more sensitive than CT to characterize subacute and chronic brain injuries,[4] but it may also depict subtle soft-tissue injuries in the acute setting, which may remain occult on CT. In this article, the authors provide a cursory review of intracranial pathologies which may be observed in the setting of TBI and provide a perspective on how MR imaging may aid in the management of patients in this setting.

Imaging Technique

The routinely acquired MR imaging sequences are often sufficient to demonstrate most TBIs. Standard pulse sequences used in most centers[7,8] for TBI imaging consist of conventional T1-weighted imaging (T1WI), T2-weighted imaging (T2WI), T2W fluid-attenuated inversion recovery (FLAIR), diffusion-weighted imaging (DWI), and a hemosiderin sensitive sequence (T2*), either

[a] Department of Radiology, Radio-Oncology and Nuclear Medicine Faculty of Medicine, University of Montréal, Montréal, QC, Canada; [b] Interventional Neuroradiology Clinical Fellow at St. Michael's Hospital, University of Toronto, Toronto, ON, Canada; [c] Department of Radiology, Centre Hospitalier de l'Université de Montréal (CHUM), 1051 Sanguinet Street, Montréal, QC H2X 0C1, Canada; [d] Department of Medical Imaging, University of Toronto, Toronto, ON, Canada
* Corresponding author. Department of Radiology, Sunnybrook Health Sciences Centre, 2075 Bayview Avenue, Toronto, ON, M4N 3M5.
E-mail address: matylda.machnowska@sunnybrook.ca

Neuroimag Clin N Am 33 (2023) 235–249
https://doi.org/10.1016/j.nic.2022.12.001
1052-5149/23/Crown Copyright © 2023 Published by Elsevier Inc. All rights reserved.

Table 1
MR signal of intracranial blood products

	Delay	Hemoglobin Degradation Status	T1WI	T2WI	T2*
Hyperacute	<6 h	Oxyhemoglobin	Mild hyperintense	Very hyperintense	Peripheral hypointensity
Late acute	6–72 h	Deoxyhemoglobin	Isointense to hypointense	hypointense	Hypointense (blooming)
Early subacute	3 days to 1 week	Intracellular methemoglobin	Very hyperintense	Hypointense	Hypointense (blooming)
Late subacute	1–2 weeks to 2 months	Extracellular methemoglobin	Very hyperintense	Very hyperintense (with peripheral hypointensity)	Variable
Chronic	2 weeks to years	Hemosiderin	Hypointense	Hypointense	Hypointense (blooming)

susceptibility-weighted imaging (SWI) or gradient-recalled echo (GRE) imaging.

Indication

TBI can be subcategorized according to timing of injury (acute: 0–7 days; subacute: 8–89 days; and chronic: more than 90 days later)[7,9] and severity of injury (mild: Glasgow Coma Scale [GCS] of 13–15; moderate: GCS of 9–12; and severe: GCS of 3–8).[10–12] Although head CT is usually appropriate as the initial imaging in moderate to severe head trauma, as well as in mild head trauma if indicated by clinical findings,brain MRI may be appropriate as the short-term follow-up imaging in acute head trauma if there are positive findings on CT.[9] In subacute or chronic head trauma with unexplained cognitive or neurologic deficits, both CT and MR imaging head are usually appropriate. MR angiography (MRA) and MR venography (MRV) may also be appropriate when there are clinical risk factors or positive findings on prior imaging for arterial or venous injury, as an alternative to CT angiography (CTA) and CT venography (CTV). .

INTRA-AXIAL TRAUMA
Contusions

Imaging findings/pathology

Contusions are the most common form of intra-axial injury. They are most often due to blunt closed head trauma, which causes brain tissue to impact against the skull or dural reflections (falx cerebri and tentorium cerebelli).[13] Rarely, open head trauma, such as depressed skull fractures, may also result in contusions of the impacted brain parenchyma. Hemorrhagic components are common and the MR signal depends on timing of injury (Table 1).[14]

Contusions always involve the superficial areas of the brain, but more severe impact injuries, often termed cerebral lacerations, may also involve the deep white matter and basal ganglia (Box 1). The most affected areas are the temporal poles, peri-sylvian gyri, and orbitofrontal lobes (Fig. 1). The occipital poles are the least commonly affected areas, but may be involved as "contrecoup" injuries, which represent contusions that occur at 180° from the point of impact, or "coup" lesions. They are often accompanied by subarachnoid hemorrhage (discussed further below).

Clinical applications

In the typical clinical setting, most contusions will be detected on CT, and follow-up imaging will be based on the severity of imaging findings (small cortical contusion or small intraparenchymal hemorrhage ≤10 mL) and clinical status of the patient.[15] However, depending on timing of imaging, the initial CT evaluation may be negative[16] or it may underestimate the true extent of associated soft tissue injury.[17] In fact, about half

Box 1
Differential Diagnosis for contusions

- Diffuse axonal injury (DAI): Contusions predominantly involve the superficial areas of the brain, with significant cortical involvement, whereas DAI usually shows cortical sparing.

- Brain laceration: Actual laceration of the pial membrane characterized by extension of hemorrhage to the deep white matter/basal ganglia. A full thickness laceration may extend from the cortex to the ventricle.

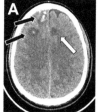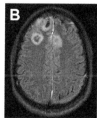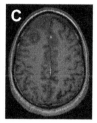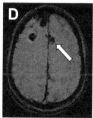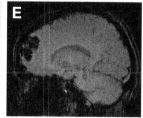

Fig. 1. (*A*) Axial noncontrast CT (NCCT) demonstrates bifrontal hemorrhagic (*black arrows*) and nonhemorrhagic contusions (*white arrow*). MR imaging better demonstrates true extent of injury on FLAIR (*B*). T1WI (*C*) and SWI (*D* and *E*) reveal hemorrhagic component within the left frontal paramedian contusion, which was occult on CT (*white arrow*).

of patients will demonstrate some degree of radiological progression in the first 24 to 48 hours, and up to 20% of initially conservatively managed patients will present hematoma expansion with mass effect on follow-up, requiring surgery.[18] MR imaging is more sensitive than CT for detecting hemorrhagic and nonhemorrhagic portions of cerebral contusions,[19,20] especially when contusions are located near the calvarium and during the acute phase of TBI, when there is still minimal edema (Fig. 2). However, studies have found that such findings usually do not lead to change in acute management,[21] but may be of use regarding prognostication of patients.[22–25]

Diffuse Axonal Injury

Imaging findings/pathology
DAI is mostly seen in the context of high velocity trauma, such as motor vehicle accidents, where brain tissues are submitted to rapid acceleration/deceleration. The resulting inertial forces applied to the cortex, white matter, and deep gray nuclei, which all move at different speed, cause stretching, and subsequent lysis of axons, characterized by cytotoxic edema on imaging.[26,27] Severe trauma may also cause tearing of the penetrating

vessels along the white matter, resulting in punctate hemorrhage/microhemorrhage, a phenomenon termed diffuse vascular injury.[27,28]

Axonal injuries are most often seen at areas of intersection between gray and white matter, such as the subcortical white matter, most often anteriorly, as well as areas of dense white matter tracts, such as the corpus callosum and in the midbrain/upper pons, characterized as punctate areas of increased T2/FLAIR signal (Box 2). The pathological grading of DAI[29] was ported to imaging by Gentry and colleagues,[5] with stage 1 consisting of lobar involvement, stage 2 callosal involvement, and stage 3 brainstem involvement. Various studies have attempted to evaluate prognostic validity of imaging staging of DAI, with varying results,[30–33] and some have proposed more novel classifications, including one underlining the importance of substantia nigra involvement.[30]

Clinical applications
Extensive DAI may go undetected on CT, especially if there is little to no hemorrhagic component, but will most often be readily detected on a standard unenhanced brain MR imaging (Fig. 3). MR imaging also demonstrates higher sensitivity for

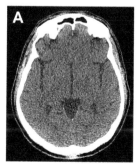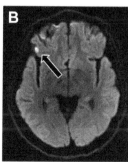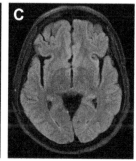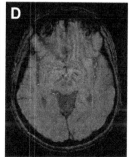

Fig. 2. (*A*) Axial NCCT in blunt head trauma fails to demonstrate subtle nonhemorrhagic right frontal contusion, only seen on axial DWI sequence (*B, black arrow*), with little to no correlation on axial FLAIR (*C*) and SWI (*D*) sequences.

Box 2
Differential Diagnosis for DAI

- Cortical contusions: DAI typically spares the overlying cortex but may coexist with cortical contusions.
- Chronic small vessel ischemic disease: Predominantly involves deep white matter, whereas DAI has a stronger predilection for subcortical white matter and corpus callosum. DAI may have hemorrhagic component on T2* sequences.
- Cerebral fat embolism: Context of displaced long bone fracture and associated symptoms of hypoxia and/or petechial skin rash.
- Cerebral amyloid angiopathy and microbleeds of the chronically ill: Diffuse pattern and mostly microhemorrhagic, whereas DAI has a more subcortical pattern and also demonstrates nonhemorrhagic component.

microhemorrhage detection, using GRE or SWI imaging.[19] Similar to above discussion on contusions, early detection of grading of DAI injury may aid in prognostication and help guide other medical decisions regarding management of patient's subacute/chronic condition (need for rehabilitation, long-term care, tracheostomy, and so forth), but most often will not affect acute management.[21–25]

EXTRA-AXIAL TRAUMA
Epidural Hematoma

Imaging findings/pathology
Epidural hematomas (EDHs) consist of hemorrhagic collections between cranial bones and their periosteum (or outer layer of the dura). As such, they are usually limited by cranial sutures, where the periosteum typically folds around the bone, except in rare anatomical variants. If significant in size, as can be the case when the cause of hemorrhage is arterial, EDH may distend the periosteum enough to appear biconvex or lentiform (Fig. 4). However, in the minority of cases where the cause of hemorrhage is venous and where hematoma is small, the classic lentiform appearance may not be as evident on imaging. Venous EDHs may also cross suture lines.

EDH types also differ in terms of location; arterial EDHs are most often supratentorial, located along the pterion and middle cranial fossa, where direct impact and/or fracture may damage large emerging dural arterial vessels along the cranial vault and skull base, whereas venous EDHs are more often located along a fracture line crossing dural venous sinuses, most often at the level of the vertex or posterior fossa (Fig. 5).

Clinical applications
EDHs of arterial origin may increase in size, and some may require surgical decompression, although many are treated conservatively. Decision to proceed with surgery is most often based on the degree of clinical impairment and stability of hematoma on CT. As such, MR has little implications in their management. However, in terms of venous EDH, MR imaging is often more sensitive and may reveal a small hemorrhagic collections not seen on CT.

Subdural Hematoma

Imaging findings/pathology
Subdural hematomas (SDHs) are hemorrhagic collections located within the potential space between the dura and the arachnoid membrane. As such, they can layer along the skull base (especially along the middle cranial fossa) and the dural reflections (flax cerebri and tentorium cerebelli), but generally do not cross these sites of dural attachments (Box 3). They may be the result of impact or nonimpact trauma, especially when there is underlying atrophy, which may facilitate trauma to the bridging veins as they cross the subdural space to reach the dural venous sinuses. Trauma to the arachnoid membrane may cause admixture of cerebrospinal fluid (CSF) in the subarachnoid space (ie, hygroma).

Clinical applications
Large SDHs (≥10 mm), with associated with midline shift (≥5 mm) or neurological symptoms, may require surgical decompression,[34,35] whereas smaller traumatic SDH (≤10 mm) in mild TBIs may be managed conservatively. A subset of such patients (roughly 10–23%) will demonstrate progression in size of SDH on follow-up imaging, requiring surgical intervention,[35,36] especially in older patients with more acute hemorrhage and larger hematoma depth. CT is usually sufficient for diagnosis and follow-up, especially in the acute phase, but a small isodense subacute SDH may initially be missed on CT (Fig. 6). MR imaging shows higher sensitivity and specificity in diagnosing SDHs, especially in the subacute/chronic phase, and can readily distinguish hemorrhagic from nonhemorrhagic collections, such as hygromas especially on FLAIR sequence. MR imaging may also more readily identify sequelae of SDH in the late subacute/chronic phase, characterized by hypointense changes on T2* (GRE, SWI), which are often more conspicuous along dural reflections; this may be useful in patients

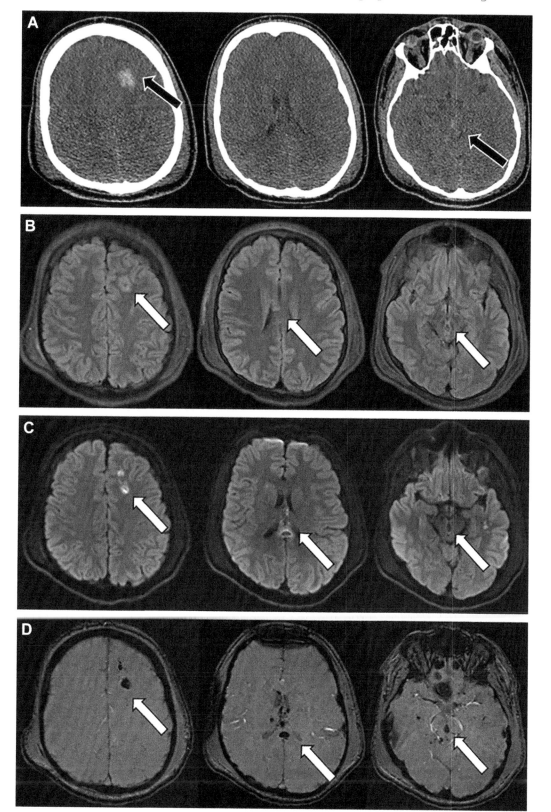

Fig. 3. Axial acquisitions at the level of the centrum semiovale (left column), corpus callosum (middle column), and midbrain (right column) on CT (*A*), MR imaging FLAIR (*B*), DWI (*C*), and SWI (*D*) demonstrate increased conspicuity of DAI on MR imaging (*white arrows*) compared with CT (*black arrows*).

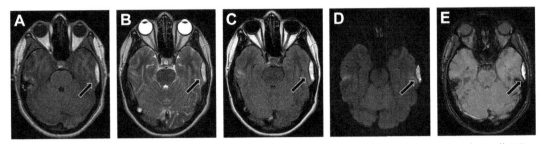

Fig. 4. Left temporal EDH of arterial origin, with biconvex appearance and hyperintense signal on all MR sequences (*black arrows*), including T1WI (*A*), T2WI (*B*), FLAIR (*C*), DWI (*D*), and SWI (*E*).

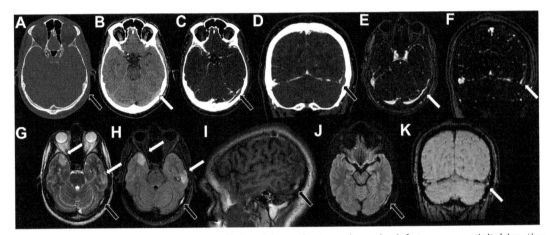

Fig. 5. Axial NCCT (*A, B*) demonstrates nondisplaced bone fracture along the left temporo-occipital junction (*black arrow*), crossing the left transverse venous sinus, with associated venous EDH (*white arrow*). Narrowing of left transverse venous sinus on CTV (*black arrow, C* and *D*). Similar findings on contrast-enhanced MRV (*white arrows, E* and *F*), with hyperintense signal of hematoma (*black arrows*) on T2WI (*G*), FLAIR (*H*), T1WI (*I*) and DWI (*J*), as well as slight peripheral blooming on SWI (*white arrow, K*). MR imaging also demonstrates bitemporal non-hemorrhagic contusions (*white arrows, G* and *H*).

Box 3
Differential Diagnosis for SDH

- EDH: Biconvex appearance, as opposed to crescent-shaped SDH. Fixed by periosteal layer of dura cannot cross suture lines but can cross dural reflections.
- Subdural hygroma: Similar in appearance to SDH, except for predominantly CSF signal (Fig. 7). The two are not mutually exclusive and a subdural collection may contain a mixture of blood and CSF.
- Contusion: Inward displacement or "buckling" of the gray matter/white matter interface can help distinguish extra-axial from intra-axial trauma.

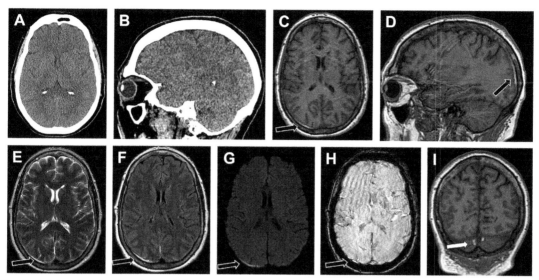

Fig. 6. Axial and sagittal NCCT (*A, B*) fail to demonstrate right occipital region small subdural hematoma, only seen on MR imaging (*black arrows*), with hyperintense signal on T1WI (*C and D*), T2WI (*E*), FLAIR (*F*), and DWI (*G*). Slight blooming can be seen at the periphery of the collection on SWI (*H*). Slight layering along the occipital sinus can also be seen on coronal T1WI (*white arrow, I*).

with unclear history of trauma and delayed presentation.

Traumatic Subarachnoid Hemorrhage

Imaging findings/pathology
Some degree of subarachnoid hemorrhage (SAH) is found in almost all cases of moderate to severe head trauma, in both impact and nonimpact types of injuries, and is usually related to tearing of small cortical vessels or underlying contusions. In most cases, blood usually collects within the sulci at the point of impact, but may extend over a significant portion of the brain in more severe injuries often associated with adjacent contusion or EDH/SDH (Box 4).

Clinical applications

- Traumatic SAH is usually managed supportively, although cases of severe SAH may require vasospasm prophylaxis. CT is usually adequate for diagnosis and follow-up of SAH, and MR imaging is rarely indicated in this context. However, MR imaging demonstrates higher detection rate than CT for small SAH,[37] especially during the subacute phase, where blood may appear isodense to CSF on CT. The lack of FLAIR signal nulling within the cerebral sulci (see Fig. 7) is an especially sensitive radiological sign of SAH in acute phase. Blooming on T2* (GRE, SWI) may be more sensitive in chronic phase.

SECONDARY BRAIN INJURY
Herniation

Imaging findings/pathology
In TBI, any focal or diffuse mass effect (brain swelling, intra-axial /extra-axial collections) may lead to herniation phenomenon. Multiple types of non-mutually exclusive herniation phenomenon can occur.

Box 4
Differential Diagnosis for traumatic SAH

- Nontraumatic SAH: Predominantly involves the basal cisterns (as opposed to the cerebral convexities) and is usually more diffuse. Underlying vascular lesion identified on CTA/MRA (most commonly an aneurysm).

- Cerebral edema: Sometimes associated with pseudosubarachnoid hemorrhage appearance on CT because of hypodense appearance of the brain compared with the relatively dense blood vessels within the subarachnoid spaces. The lack of CSF hypointensity on T2* (GRE, SWI) or hyperintensity on FLAIR can help distinguish this phenomenon from SAH.

- Other causes associated with the lack of CSF signal nulling on FLAIR (eg, meningitis, leptomeningeal carcinomatosis, supplemental oxygen therapy, recent gadolinium injection, and magnetic susceptibility artifact): History and other associated imaging findings can help distinguish from actual SAH.

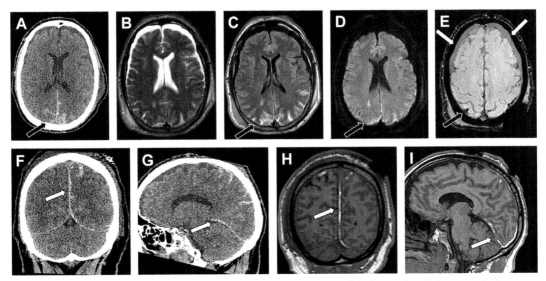

Fig. 7. Axial NCCT scan (*A*) demonstrates post-traumatic biparietal SAH (*black arrow*), which appear isointense to CSF on T2WI (*B*), but is much more conspicuous on FLAIR (*black arrow, C*) due to the lack of CSF signal nulling. There is slight hyperintensity within the sulci on DWI (*black arrow, D*), with associated blooming on SWI (*black arrow, E*) due to degrading blood products. MR imaging also better demonstrates bifrontal CSF isointense collections, displacing the cortical bridging veins on SWI (*white arrows, E*), compatible with bilateral hygromas. Coronal and sagittal NCCT (*F* and *G*) and T1WI (*H* and *I*) reveal concomitant thin subdural hematomas layering along the dural reflections (*white arrows*).

- Subfalcine:
  - Herniation of the ipsilateral ventricle and cingulate gyrus across the midline
  - May be associated with foramen of Monroe obstruction (with associated hydrocephalus) and wedging of the anterior cerebral artery (ACA) against the falx cerebri with possible ACA territory infarction.
- Descending transtentorial (Box 5):

Box 5
Differential Diagnosis for descending transtentorial herniation

- Ascending transtentroial herniation: More often seen in the oncological context (posterior fossa mass) but may be seen in cases of TBI predominantly involving the posterior fossa. Characterized by effacement of superior vermian cistern, then quadrigeminal cistern and compression of the tectal plate.

- Intracranial hypotension: Inferior displacement of brainstem and tonsils from decreased spinal CSF pressure ("brain sag" phenomenon), in cases of CSF leak.

- Chari 1 malformation: Congenital inferior displacement of tonsils, due to posterior fossa configuration, without associated supratentorial mass effect.

  - Medial displacement of ipsilateral uncus and medial temporal lobes, effacing the suprasellar and quadrigeminal cisterns, respectively.
  - May be associated with ipsilateral cranial nerve III palsy andposterior cerebral artery (PCA) infarcts, due to compression against the tentorial incisura.
- Tonsillar:
  - Inferior displacement of cerebellar tonsils, more than 5 mm below the foramen magnum, with effacement of CSF spaces at the foramen magnum and associated compression against bony margins of the foramen magnum.
  - May be associated with obstructive hydrocephalus and tonsillar necrosis.

Clinical applications
Most herniation phenomena are readily identified on CT, with the exception of tonsillar herniation, which may more conspicuous on MR imaging (as detailed above). However, MR imaging can be useful in identifying early complications related to herniation phenomenon, such as subependymal CSF resorption in early hydrocephalus, early midbrain changes in Duret hemorrhages, and herniation-related infarction phenomenon (ACA territory in subfalcine herniation, PCA territory in descending transtentorial herniation, Fig. 8).

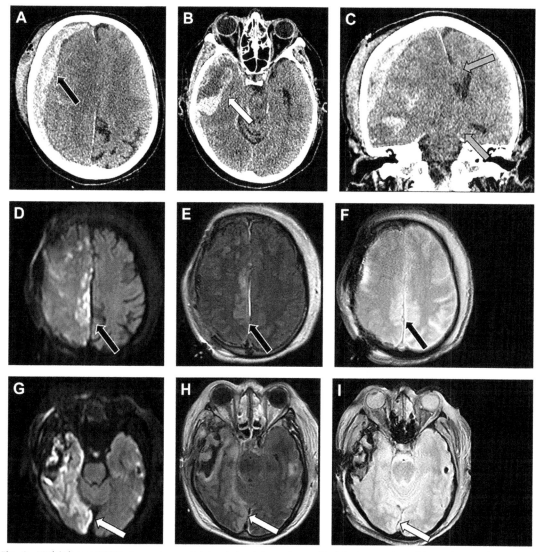

Fig. 8. Multiplanar NCCT shows large right subdural hematoma (*A, black arrow*) and large hemorrhagic right temporal contusion (*B, black arrow*), with associated mass effect, resulting in leftward subfalcine and left uncal herniation (*C, gray arrows*). MR imaging performed post-right hemicraniectomy and external ventricular drain placement showed decreased mass effect, but also revealed subacute infarcts within the right ACA (*black arrows*) and right PCA (*white arrows*) territories, best demonstrated by diffusion restriction on DWI (*D and G*), but also seen on FLAIR (*E and F*), without hemorrhagic component detected on GRE (*H and I*).

Box 6

Differential Diagnosis for ischemia

- Cerebral swelling/edema only: No significant restriction on DWI. There may be overlap in imaging findings between TBI and non-TBI cases with infarction.

Box 7

Differential Diagnosis for cerebral fat emboli

- Embolic infarcts of other cause (eg, cardiac, carotid plaque): Usually not as numerous and rarely predominantly involve white matter.

- DAI: Blooming on DAI usually more linear. Component of DAI difficult to rule out in patients with polytrauma and microhemorragic white matter abnormalities.

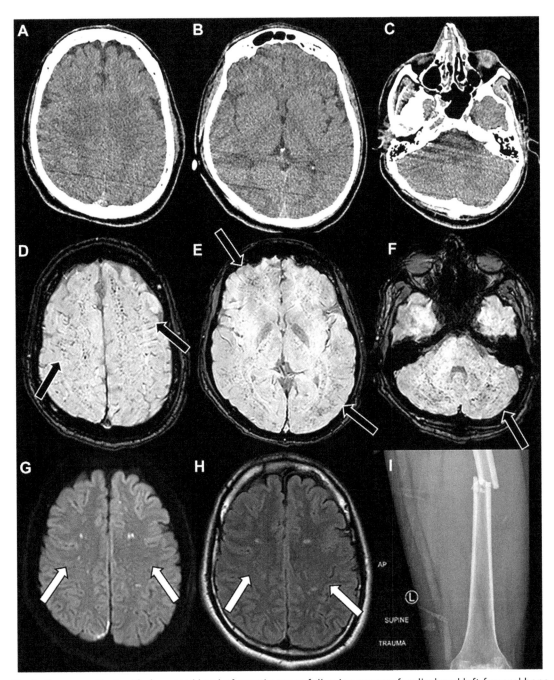

Fig. 9. Trauma patient with decreased level of consciousness following surgery for displaced left femoral bone fracture. NCCT (*A–C*) does not demonstrate any intracranial abnormality. MR imaging reveals innumerable punctate foci of increased susceptibility distributed diffusely throughout the brain, with extensive white matter involvement (*D–F, black arrows*), some of which show diffusion restriction (*G, white arrows*) and appear hyperintense on FLAIR (*H, white arrows*), suggestive of fat emboli in the clinical context of acute long bone fracture (*I*).

Ischemia/Infarction

Imaging findings/pathology

Secondary infarction in the context of TBI is most commonly related to herniation phenomenon (see

Fig. 8) but can also be related to blunt cerebrovascular injuries (eg, vascular dissection/transection or venous thrombosis), perfusion abnormalities (diffuse or focal), decreased vascular supply

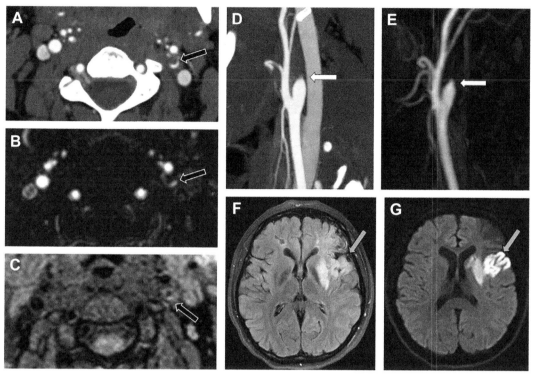

Fig. 10. Axial CTA (*A*) showing occlusion at the origin of the left ICA (*black arrows*), also demonstrated on contrast enhanced MRA of the carotids (*B*), with associated slightly T1 hyperintense signal abnormality adjacent to narrowed flow void on fat-saturated T1 sequence (*C*). Coronal reformats of the occluded proximal left cervical ICA demonstrate rat tail appearance (*white arrows*) on both CTA (*D*) and MRA (*E*). Subacute infarct in the left MCA territory (*gray arrows*) is seen on FLAIR (*F*) and DWI (*G*) sequences, likely from artery-to-artery embolic phenomenon.

(secondary to increased mass effect), and/or increased vascular demand (secondary to excitotoxic brain injury).

Clinical applications

Areas of infarction can readily be detected on CT, characterized by loss of gray–white matter interface, but conspicuity of findings often lags behind the clinical picture. In comparison, MR imaging has been shown to be more sensitive and specific in diagnosing post-traumatic infarction, especially in the acute phase, although rarely performed in this context (Box 6). Diffusion restriction is especially sensitive and predates CT changes by hours.

Cerebral Fat Emboli

Imaging findings/pathology

In the setting of displaced long bone fractures (usually in the lower extremities), embolization of fat particles in the brain results in innumerable punctate infarcts and inflammation of the surrounding brain parenchyma, often associated with petechial/hemorrhagic component. Other associated systemic findings include hypoxia

(from pulmonary emboli) and petechial rash (from immune reaction).

MR imaging findings will depend on the timing of injury,[38] with initially scattered innumerable punctate foci of T2/FLAIR hyperintense signal abnormalities with associated diffusion restriction throughout the brain in the acute phase (Box 7). Signal abnormalities may become confluent, especially in subacute phase. Atrophy and gliosis can follow during the chronic phase. Blooming can be seen on T2* sequences, representing petechial hemorrhage, present from acute to the chronic phase.

Clinical applications

The innumerable punctate infarcts of fat emboli are often inconspicuous on CT (Fig. 9), as no macroscopic fat droplets can be seen. Therefore, MR imaging is much more sensitive and specific then CT in this context and should be considered in trauma patients with displaced long bone fractures presenting neurologic dysfunction, especially when presenting without a clear history of head injury.

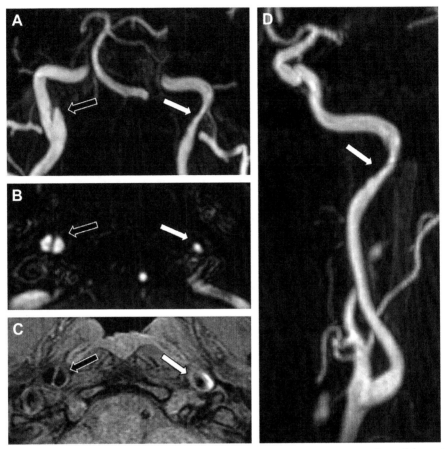

Fig. 11. Multiplanar contrast-enhanced MRA of the carotids (*A, B, D*) demonstrating bilateral dissections of the distal cervical internal carotid arteries, best appreciated on coronal plane (*A*), with pseudoaneurysm on the right (*black arrow*) and stenosis on the left (*white arrow*), the latter more conspicuous on dedicated coronal oblique reformat (*D*). Axial MRA (*B*) demonstrates asymmetry of distal cervical ICA segments caliber, narrowed on the left (*white arrow*), while an while an intimal flap is seen on the right (*black arrow*). Axial T1WI with fat saturation (*C*) demonstrates prominent T1 hyperintense crescent surrounding narrowed distal left cervical internal carotid artery flow void on the left (*white arrow*), compatible with intramural hematoma.

VASCULAR INJURIES
Craniocervical Arterial Dissection

Imaging findings/pathology

Dissections are characterized by a tear of one or more layers of the blood vessels, allowing blood to dissect in between said layers, which may stenose or occlude the vessel lumen, or even result in outpouchings called pseudoaneurysms, which can rupture. Imaging on MR imaging may show pathognomonic collection of blood product of various age along the afflicted blood vessel (classically crescent-shaped in appearance, as shown in Figs. 10 and 11), which may only appear as a vague vessel wall thickening on CT/CTA (Box 8). Dissections may be associated with artery-to-artery embolism, resulting in infarcts within the distal territory of the afflicted artery, best seen on DWI.

Craniocervical arterial dissections can be intracranial and extracranial and are most often located where blood vessels transition from a fixed to a mobile segment. The cervical internal carotid

---

Box 8
Differential Diagnosis for craniocervical arterial dissection

- Atherosclerosis: More often involves origin of the great vessels and carotid bifurcation. Intracranially, may involve multiple vascular territory. May be assessed more accurately on vessel wall MR imaging.

- Vasospasm: Self-resolving process on repeat imaging; extracranial involvement: absence of flap or intramural hematoma; and intracranial involvement: distribution in multiple vascular territories.

artery (ICA) is the most common location, often just below the petrous canal, followed by the V3 segment of the vertebral arteries (between C1 and C2). Traumatic intracranial dissections most commonly involve the V4 segments of the vertebral arteries.

Clinical applications

Extracranial arterial dissections most often present a benign natural history, with high rates of resolution/recanalization, and are usually managed conservatively. However, early recognition is key,

as timely antiplatelet/anticoagulation therapy may prevent serious ischemic complications secondary to artery-to-artery embolism. As such, the increased sensitivity and specificity of MR imaging in detecting dissections may prove useful in this context.

Although management of intracranial dissections remains controversial, the advent of vessel-wall imaging using MR imaging has proven useful in diagnosing this previously underrecognized pathology.

Dural Venous Sinus Thrombosis

Imaging findings/pathology

Thrombosis within the dural venous sinuses may be seen directly as a filling defect on MRV, or indirectly as peri-sinus parenchymal edema due to venous congestion, which can progress to cytotoxic edema, with diffusion restriction from venous infarct, or can be associated with parenchymal hemorrhagic transformation (Box 9. In the context of trauma, dural venous thrombosis is most often found when a skull fracture crosses a dural venous sinus or the jugular bulb (Fig. 12).

Clinical applications

Trauma represents only one of the many causes of dural sinus thrombosis (roughly 1.1%).[39] Other, far more prevalent causes include oral contraceptive use, pregnant/puerperal status, hypercoagulable state, and infection. Nevertheless, in patients with skull fractures extending to the dural sinus or jugular bulb, venous imaging with CT venogram

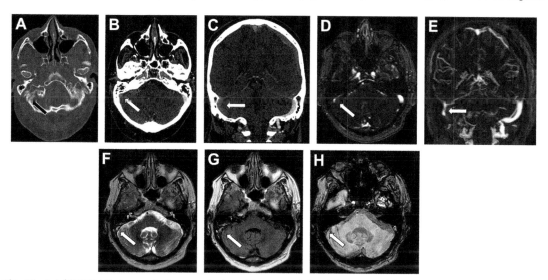

Fig. 12. Axial NCCT (A) demonstrates nondisplaced fracture of the right occipital bone (black arrow), adjacent to the right jugular bulb and right distal sigmoid sinus, which appears hyperdense and fails to enhance on CTV (B and C, white arrows). Phase-contrast MRV also demonstrates the lack of enhancement within the sigmoid sinus and right jugular bulb (D and E, white arrows), with associated lack of flow void on T2WI (F) and FLAIR (G) and slight blooming on SWI (H), more evident when compared with contralateral sigmoid sinus.

(CTV) or MRV is recommended. Venous sinus thrombosis in trauma patients represent a clinical challenge, as caretakers must weigh between the risk of thrombosis progression and the risk of exacerbated hemorrhage (intracranial or otherwise) with anticoagulation. As such, repeated imaging may be necessary in order to ensure stability of clot extent. A few studies have compared the accuracy of CTV with MRV and have found similar sensitivity and specificity.[40,41] Despite increased ease of access and better evaluation of bony findings on CTV, MRV may represent a useful adjunct in trauma patient undergoing frequent follow-up when attempting to delay anticoagulation, given concern for radiation exposure with repeated CT examinations.

SUMMARY

MR imaging has been shown to have higher sensitivity than CT for traumatic intracranial soft tissue injuries, as well as most cases of intracranial hemorrhage, thus making it a significant adjunct to CT in the management of TBI, mostly in the subacute to chronic phase, but also in the acute phase, when there are persistent neurologic symptoms unexplained by CT imaging. Although CT remains the modality of choice in most cases of acute TBI because of ease of access, faster imaging time, lower imaging cost, and better sensitivity for concomitant bony injuries, significant developments in image acquisition strategies have enabled more widespread use of MR imaging in the acute and subacute phases of TBI, yielding relevant data for long-term decision-making and prognostication efforts.

DISCLOSURE

The Authors have nothing to disclose.

REFERENCES

1. Reid LD, Fingar KR. Inpatient Stays and Emergency Department Visits Involving Traumatic Brain Injury, 2017. 2020 Mar 31. In: Healthcare Cost and Utilization Project (HCUP) Statistical Briefs [Internet]. Rockville (MD): Agency for Healthcare Research and Quality (US); 2006 Feb-. Statistical Brief #255.
2. Taylor CA, Bell JM, Breiding MJ, et al. Traumatic Brain Injury–Related Emergency Department Visits, Hospitalizations, and Deaths — United States, 2007 and 2013. MMWR Surveill Summ 2017;66(9): 1–16.
3. Centers for Disease Control and Prevention National Center for Health Statistics: Mortality data on CDC WONDER, Available at: https://wonder.cdc.gov/mcd.html. Accessed July 15, 2022.
4. Davis PC. Expert Panel on Neurologic Imaging Head trauma. AJNR Am J Neuroradiol 2007;28(8): 1619–21.
5. Gentry LR. Imaging of closed head injury. Radiology 1994;191(1):1–17.
6. Quaday KA, Salzman JG, Gordon BD. Magnetic resonance imaging and computed tomography utilization trends in an academic. Am J Emerg Med 2014;32(6):524–8.
7. Wintermark M, Sanelli PC, Anzai Y, et al. Imaging Evidence and Recommendations for Traumatic Brain Injury: Conventional Neuroimaging Techniques. J Am Coll Radiol 2015;12(2):e1–14.
8. Lee AL. Advanced Imaging of Traumatic Brain Injury. Korean J Neurotrauma 2020;16. https://doi.org/10.13004/kjnt.2020.16.e12.
9. Shih RY, Burns J, Ajam AA, et al. ACR Appropriateness Criteria® Head Trauma: 2021 Update. J Am Coll Radiol 2021;18(5):S13–36.
10. Grant L, Iverson MRLS. Prevalence of abnormal CT-scans following mild head injury. Brain Inj 2000; 14(12):1057–61.
11. Cushman JG, Agarwal N, Fabian TC, et al. Practice management guidelines for the management of mild traumatic brain injury: the EAST practice management guidelines work group. J Trauma 2001;51(5): 1016–26.
12. Servadei F, Teasdale G, Merry G, Neurotraumatology Committee of the World Federation of Neurosurgical S. Defining acute mild head injury in adults: a proposal based on prognostic factors, diagnosis, and management. J Neurotrauma 2001;18(7):657–64.
13. Osborn AG, Hedlund GL, Salzman KL, Concannon KE. In: Anne G. Osborn, editor, Osborn's brain: imaging, pathology, and anatomy, 2nd ed., 2017, Elsevier, Salt Lake, 488.
14. Yousem DM, Grossman RI. Neuroradiology: the requisites. Philadelphia, PA: Mosby/Elsevier; 2010.
15. Washington CW, Grubb RL Jr. Are routine repeat imaging and intensive care unit admission necessary in mild traumatic brain injury? J Neurosurg 2012; 116(3):549–57.
16. Turcato G, Cipriano A, Zaboli A, et al. Risk of delayed intracranial haemorrhage after an initial negative CT in patients on DOACs with mild traumatic brain injury. Am J Emerg Med 2022;53:185–9.
17. Kurland D, Hong C, Aarabi B, et al. Hemorrhagic Progression of a Contusion after Traumatic Brain Injury: A Review. J Neurotrauma 2012;29(1):19–31.
18. Alahmadi H, Vachhrajani S, Cusimano MD. The natural history of brain contusion: an analysis of radiological and clinical progression. J Neurosurg 2010; 112(5):1139–45.
19. Amyot F, Arciniegas DB, Brazaitis MP, et al. A Review of the Effectiveness of Neuroimaging Modalities for the Detection of Traumatic Brain Injury. J Neurotrauma 2015;32(22):1693–721.

20. Schweitzer AD, Niogi SN, Whitlow CT, et al. Traumatic Brain Injury: Imaging Patterns and Complications. Radiographics 2019;39(6):1571–95.

21. Manolakaki D, Velmahos GC, Spaniolas K, et al. Early magnetic resonance imaging is unnecessary in patients with traumatic brain injury. J Trauma 2009;66(4):1008–12 [discussion: 1012-4].

22. Richter S, Winzeck S, Kornaropoulos EN, et al. Neuroanatomical Substrates and Symptoms Associated With Magnetic Resonance Imaging of Patients With Mild Traumatic Brain Injury. JAMA Netw Open 2021;4(3):e210994.

23. Yuh EL, Mukherjee P, Lingsma HF, et al. Magnetic resonance imaging improves 3-month outcome prediction in mild traumatic brain injury. Ann Neurol 2013;73(2):224–35.

24. Massaad E, Shin JH, Gibbs WN. The Prognostic Role of Magnetic Resonance Imaging Biomarkers in Mild Traumatic Injury. JAMA Netw Open 2021; 4(3):e211824.

25. Haghbayan H, Boutin A, Laflamme M, et al. The Prognostic Value of MRI in Moderate and Severe Traumatic Brain Injury: A Systematic Review and Meta-Analysis. Crit Care Med 2017;45(12):e1280–8.

26. Vo DT, Phan CC, Le HGN, et al. Diffuse axonal injury: a case report and MRI findings. Radiol Case Rep 2022;17(1):91–4.

27. Haber M, Amyot F, Lynch CE, et al. Imaging biomarkers of vascular and axonal injury are spatially distinct in chronic traumatic brain injury. J Cereb Blood Flow Metab 2021;41(8):1924–38.

28. Iwamura A, Taoka T, Fukusumi A, et al. Diffuse vascular injury: convergent-type hemorrhage in the supratentorial white matter on susceptibility-weighted image in cases of severe traumatic brain damage. Neuroradiology 2012;54(4):335–43.

29. Adams JH, Doyle D, Ford I, et al. Diffuse axonal injury in head injury: Definition, diagnosis and grading. Histopathology 1989;15(1):49–59.

30. Abu Hamdeh S, Marklund N, Lannsjo M, et al. Extended Anatomical Grading in Diffuse Axonal Injury Using MRI: Hemorrhagic Lesions in the Substantia Nigra and Mesencephalic Tegmentum Indicate Poor Long-Term Outcome. J Neurotrauma 2017;34(2):341–52.

31. Van Eijck MM, Schoonman GG, Van Der Naalt J, et al. Diffuse axonal injury after traumatic brain injury is a prognostic factor for functional outcome: a systematic review and meta-analysis. Brain Inj 2018; 32(4):395–402.

32. Van Eijck MM, Herklots MW, Peluso J, et al. Accuracy in prediction of long-term functional outcome in patients with traumatic axonal injury: a comparison of MRI scales. Brain Inj 2020;34(5):595–601.

33. Bruggeman GF, Haitsma IK, Dirven CMF, et al. Traumatic axonal injury (TAI): definitions, pathophysiology and imaging—a narrative review. Acta Neurochirurgica 2021;163(1):31–44.

34. Sharma R, Rocha E, Pasi M, et al. Subdural Hematoma: Predictors of Outcome and a Score to Guide Surgical Decision-Making. J Stroke Cerebrovasc Dis 2020;29(11):105180.

35. Lee JJ, Won Y, Yang T, et al. Risk Factors of Chronic Subdural Hematoma Progression after Conservative Management of Cases with Initially Acute Subdural Hematoma. Korean J Neurotrauma 2015;11(2):52.

36. Son S, Yoo CJ, Lee SG, et al. Natural Course of Initially Non-Operated Cases of Acute Subdural Hematoma : The Risk Factors of Hematoma Progression. J Korean Neurosurg Soc 2013;54(3):211.

37. Verma RK, Kottke R, Andereggen L, et al. Detecting subarachnoid hemorrhage: Comparison of combined FLAIR/SWI versus CT. Eur J Radiol 2013; 82(9):1539–45.

38. Kuo KH, Pan YJ, Lai YJ, et al. Dynamic MR Imaging Patterns of Cerebral Fat Embolism: A Systematic Review with Illustrative Cases. Am J Neuroradiology 2014;35(6):1052–7.

39. Ferro JM, Canhao PC, Stam J, et al. Prognosis of Cerebral Vein and Dural Sinus Thrombosis. Stroke 2004;35(3):664–70.

40. Ozsvath RR, Casey SO, Lustrin ES, et al. Cerebral venography: comparison of CT and MR projection venography. AJR Am J Roentgenol 1997;169(6): 1699–707.

41. Khandelwal N, Agarwal A, Kochhar R, et al. Comparison of CT venography with MR venography in cerebral sinovenous thrombosis. AJR Am J Roentgenol 2006;187(6):1637–43.

Conventional MR Imaging in Trauma Management in Pediatrics

Helen M. Branson, BSc, MBBS, FRANZCR[a],*, Claudia Martinez-Rios, MD[a,b]

KEYWORDS

- Pediatrics • Magnetic resonance imaging • Traumatic brain injury • Diffuse axonal injury
- Contusion • Susceptibility weighted imaging

KEY POINTS

- Imaging of acute pediatric traumatic brain injury almost universally starts with computed tomography (CT) primarily due to ease of use and rapidity and often without the need for sedation.
- Magnetic Resonance (MR) imaging is more sensitive at detecting parenchymal injury that can be CT occult.
- MR imaging is advantageous in the setting where initial CT imaging is normal but abnormal neurological symptoms persist.
- Conventional MR imaging can be achieved with a fast protocol in the acute emergency setting or with a longer protocol for prognosis and more detailed imaging of parenchymal injury.
- MR imaging has a low sensitivity for non-displaced fractures.

INTRODUCTION

Discussion of Problem/Clinical Presentation

Traumatic brain injury (TBI) is the major cause of death and disability in children across the world.[1-3] According to the Canadian TBI research consortium, TBI is the leading cause of death in the first half of life and contributes to chronic disability for Canadians at every age.[4] Based on data from the United States and Europe,[5] it is estimated that there are approximately 150,000 emergency room visits and hospital admissions every year due to TBI, and in Canada approximately 500,000 people are living with TBI-related disability.[4]

The aim of initial trauma management of pediatric patients is to diagnose the extent of TBI and to determine if urgent or emergent neurosurgical intervention is required. Computed tomography (CT) scans are widely available in most pediatric hospitals, and CT has been and still is the first line of investigation during the first 24 hours after injury. According to Wintermark and colleagues,[6] there is strong consensus and evidence that a noncontrast CT (NCCT) is the first recommended diagnostic imaging choice for all patients with acute moderate to severe TBI.

For more than 30 years, studies have however demonstrated a role for Magnetic Resonance (MR) imaging in assessment of the extent and location of hemorrhagic and non-hemorrhagic brain injury,[7,8] thus adding to prognostication (Fig. 1).

Why then has MR imaging not become the first line of investigation in pediatric TBI assessment on a worldwide scale? This article outlines current use of conventional MR imaging in the management of pediatric TBI.

No disclosures.
[a] Department of Diagnostic Imaging, SickKids, University of Toronto, 555 University Avenue, Toronto, Ontario M5G1X8, Canada; [b] Department of Medical Imaging, CHEO, University of Ottawa, 401 Smyth Road, Ottawa, Ontario K1H 8L1, Canada
* Corresponding author.
E-mail address: helen.branson@sickkids.ca

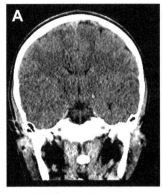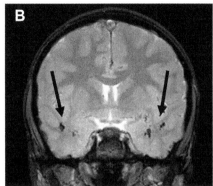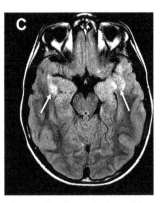

Fig. 1. (*A*) Coronal non-contrast CT shows poor definition of temporal punctate hemorrhagic contusions. These are easier to define on (*B*) coronal MPGR (*black arrows*) and (*C*) axial FLAIR (*white arrows*).

ANATOMICAL AND DEVELOPMENTAL CONSIDERATIONS IN CHILDREN

TBI in children presents challenges including difficulty in obtaining a good clinical examination (particularly in younger children) and incomplete or unknown details of the traumatic event, including timing and mechanism of injury.

The type and extent of the pediatric head trauma also varies according to patients' age,[9] due to the following:

a. Mechanism and type of trauma
b. Characteristics of the head and skull, face and brain size and anatomy
c. Brain functional development
d. Extent, pattern, and distribution of the traumatic injury

The age and development of the child will affect the type and mechanism of TBI. The following defines the most common causes of trauma in different age groups.

1. Newborns—birth-related traumatic injuries with small subdural hemorrhages along the falx/tentorium and scalp and cephalic hematomas.[1,9]
2. Toddlers—commonly suffer from falls and accidental head injury, as they become mobile.
3. School-age children—undergo TBI due to increased mobility or transportation, including riding a bicycle or car-pedestrian injury.
4. Adolescents—suffer injuries often due to motor vehicle accidents (MVA) and is a common cause of death in this age group.[9] Bicycle and sports-related accidents are also frequent especially when helmets are not worn.[1]
5. TBI secondary to nonaccidental injury (NAI) can be seen in children with a median age of 2 to 4 months,[9] with an approximate risk for hospitalization secondary to NAI in children younger than 1 year of about 30/100,000.[9,10] NAI injuries

include skull fractures, subdural hemorrhages (SDH), diffuse axonal injury (DAI), and hypoxic-ischemic injury.

There are several important anatomic considerations for TBI in children, including head size and weight, skull characteristics, open sutures, craniofacial ratio, and the immature developing brain.

- *Head size and weight*: the ratio of head to body size is largest at birth and declines with increasing age. Newborns and young infants have larger heavier heads compared with the rest of the body, making them more susceptible to TBI due to the dynamics of head acceleration and deceleration during trauma. Boys undergo approximately a 40% increase in head circumference between birth and 2 years of age.[9]
- *Skull characteristics*: distinct characteristics of the pediatric skull include patent and developing sutures and the higher plasticity of the skull, which allow better withstanding of traumatic forces. Evidence for this plasticity can be seen with the higher prevalence of the inverted "ping pong" skull fractures. The pediatric skull is more flexible with better capability to absorb impact during a traumatic event contributed also by unfused sutures.[7] The high plasticity of the skull can result in increased shear forces on the brain parenchyma with tearing and stretching between the skull, dura, vessels, and the brain, causing DAI involving the gray-white matter junction, and injury to subdural vessels, causing SDH.[7,9]
- *Open sutures*: allow for movement between the skull bones.[11] They prevent acute elevation of intracranial pressure related to edema/mass effect from intracranial collections, potentially limiting or delaying secondary injuries; this also allows propagation of cerebrospinal fluid

(CSF) pulsations along the sutures or fracture sites.[9]

- *Craniofacial ratio*: newborns and small children have a smaller face with respect to the cranium, making them increasingly susceptible to skull, rather than facial trauma. The proportion of face-cranium is 1 to 8 at birth, 1 to 4 by 5 years, and 1 to 2.5 during adolescence.[9]

- *Brain characteristics*: the brain also undergoes anatomic and functional changes over time. The newborn brain is poorly myelinated with higher water content and less cytoskeleton, compared to adults, making it softer and more prone to acceleration-deceleration injury.[9] The degree of myelination affects the absorption pattern of trauma-related forces, with higher susceptibility of the unmyelinated brain to the TBI with shear injuries. Margulies and Thibault studied the mechanisms of TBI in children and the implications on the brain compared with adults, and found that the 1-month-old infant brain and skull suffered increased distortion and changes after a direct force impact.[12]

- *Cervical spine and neck musculature*: young children have less support of their neck, and their craniocervical junction (CCJ) stability depends on the ligaments, rather than the bones. This, together with the disproportionately large head, results in higher incidence of CCJ injury. CCJ must always be assessed during TBI.[1,9] Retroclival epidural hemorrhages and tectorial membrane injury can be seen with TBI and most commonly with MVA or NAI in infants.[9,13]

DISCUSSION OF IMAGING MODALITIES IN TRAUMATIC BRAIN INJURY
Computed Tomography

CT has traditionally been recommended as the first-line investigation in pediatric TBI, as it can be performed in minutes and often does not require sedation, or if some sedation is needed it can be given by most emergency physicians. CT is widely available and cost-effective, compared with MR imaging.[14,15] The objective of CT is to promptly identify evidence and extent of structural damage and to identify findings that require immediate surgical intervention (e.g. large epidural hematomas).

Limitations of NCCT include inadequate visualization of DAI, limited visualization of non-hemorrhagic lesions and subtle parenchymal contusions, early signs of increased intracranial pressure, and small extra-axial hemorrhages or lesions in critical locations such as the corpus callosum, brainstem and cerebellar tonsils (Figs. 1-4;6).[16,17] Beam hardening from bone, metallic

objects, or calcifications can also obscure findings. Good visualization of the posterior fossa structures may be poor, making assessment limited for retroclival hematomas or cerebellar injuries. Use of ionizing radiation is also a consideration, particularly in the pediatric population. CT does, however, provide detailed imaging of the skull and face for assessment of fractures.

Conventional MR Imaging

MR imaging is not routinely used as a first line of imaging in pediatric TBI. More common indications include the following:

1. After a normal or near-normal CT but persistent neurologic symptoms
2. If there is clinical deterioration
3. To follow up on documented CT abnormalities
4. For guiding ongoing management decisions
5. For prognostication

Conventional MR imaging can be used 48 to 72 hours after injury to guide aggressive management (eg, in case of expanding intracranial hematoma requiring evacuation) and to prevent secondary brain injury. Advantages of MR imaging include improved detection of hematomas as blood products degrade, better evaluation of hemorrhagic cortical contusions, detection of shear injury with abnormal white matter signal (Figs. 1-4, 6), and detection of DAI or mild neuronal injury. MR imaging also provides better visualization of brainstem, basal ganglia, and thalami.

Limitations include accessibility, the need for general anesthesia, the long image acquisition time compared with CT, and potential external devices not compatible or safe with MR imaging (eg, external fixation devices).

In the acute setting of TBI, MR imaging can provide important information compared with CT but has failed to demonstrate significant additional findings that could change immediate management. In the chronic setting of TBI, MR imaging can be used to identify late complications, guide management, and predict long-term prognosis/outcome.[13,18]

CLINICAL APPLICATIONS OF CONVENTIONAL MR IMAGING IN TRAUMATIC BRAIN INJURY

It has long been known that MR imaging has higher sensitivity and specificity in detecting and characterizing brain changes related to traumatic injury at a higher contrast resolution, including detection of small non-hemorrhagic lesions,[8] or in the assessment of brain cortical contusions.

Hesselink and colleagues[19] studied 98 brain contusions in 17 patients aged 2 to 51 years with

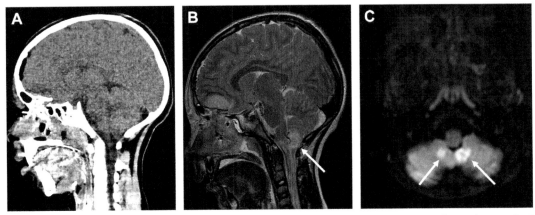

Fig. 2. (*A*) Sagittal non-contrast CT shows low densities in the inferior frontal lobe and no definite abnormality in the posterior fossa, but there is artifact at the foramen magnum. (*B*) Sagittal T2 and (*C*) axial DWI demonstrate hemorrhagic contusions with restricted diffusion in the bilateral cerebellar tonsils (*white arrows*) and edema in the inferior frontal lobe and facial trauma.

MR imaging and CT, and MR imaging showed higher sensitivity in detecting 98% of brain contusions, as compared with 56% with CT. The investigators determined that although CT was very effective for the evaluation of acute head trauma, MR imaging remained as their recommended imaging modality for complete evaluation of traumatic brain lesions.[19]

Kara and colleagues[20] prospectively studied 124 patients aged 15 to 70 years with normal head CT, but persisting neurological deficits, who underwent a repeat CT and MR imaging within the second and tenth post-traumatic day, from a cohort of 3000 patients with severe traumatic head injury, and a Glasgow Coma Scale (GCS) score equal to or less than 10. The most common lesions found in their cohort were shear injuries, cortical contusions, brainstem lesions, rare subcortical grey matter lesions, and an isolated traumatic aneurysm. The investigators highlighted the advantage of MR imaging in detecting acute and subacute hemorrhagic and non-hemorrhagic lesions and brainstem injuries, and the improved detection and delineation of parenchymal traumatic lesions, allowing a more precise diagnosis, guiding medical therapy, and estimating

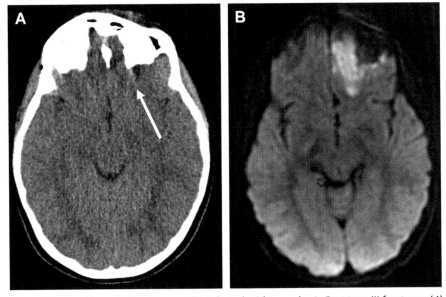

Fig. 3. Patient was involved in an ATV rollover and intubated with complex LeFort type III fractures. (*A*) Axial non-contrast CT shows mild edema and small hyperdense foci involving the left frontal lobe (*white arrow*). MRI performed 3 days later. (*B*) Axial DWI shows more extensive frontal lobes contusions with restricted diffusion.

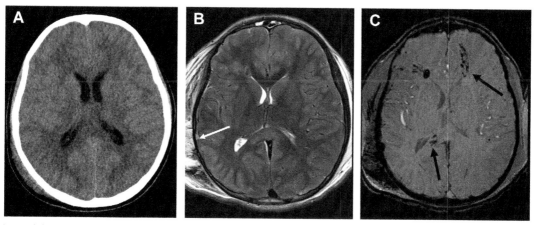

Fig. 4. (*A*) Axial non-contrast CT shows a small right parietal subgaleal hematoma and subtle effacement of the extra-axial CSF spaces and sulci. MR imaging performed 3 days later. (*B*) Axial T2 and (*C*) axial SWI demonstrate small right parietal extra-axial hemorrhage (*white arrow*), larger scalp hematoma, edema of bilateral frontal lobes, high T2 signal right parietal lobe, right thalamus and splenium of the corpus callosum, and susceptibility artifact (*black arrows*) in keeping with diffuse axonal injury.

prognosis.[20] Lindberg and colleagues[21] also highlighted the utility of MR imaging to predict prognosis and outcomes and ability to identify changes that may lead to neurodegeneration.

Conventional MR Imaging Techniques in Traumatic Brain Injury

1. *FAST MR imaging without sedation*—fast MR is an imaging protocol tailored to provide robust imaging findings of the brain using shorter acquisition times (Fig. 5). It has been used with encouraging results; however, it is not yet endorsed as the standard of care.[17]

Mehta and colleagues[21] studied 103 pediatric patients between 0 and 19 years of age presenting with acute head trauma and demonstrated that when comparing CT with rapid MR imaging, there were similar detection rates for extra-axial hemorrhage, but only moderate agreement between MR imaging and CT for hemorrhagic contusions/intra-parenchymal hemorrhage.[22]

Young and colleagues compared the detection rates for intracranial injury of fast MR imaging versus CT in 33 children aged between 3 days and 6 years presenting with acute head trauma. Thirty of thirty-three patients had identified traumatic injuries, with an overall agreement of 82% between the 2 modalities. MR imaging had a higher detection rate of epidural and subdural hematomas, subarachnoid hemorrhage, and parenchymal injuries, with 14 out of 21 skull fractures being missed.[23]

Lindberg and colleagues performed a prospective study of 223 relatively stable children younger than 6 years who sustained TBI and underwent NCCT without sedation and fast MR imaging. When using NCCT, the investigators found TBI in 111 children, missing subdural hematoma, parenchymal contusions, and subarachnoid hemorrhage. They found TBI in 103 children when using fast MR imaging, missing 0 isolated skull fractures and 2 isolated subarachnoid hemorrhages. The fast MR imaging sequences included

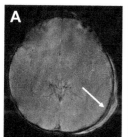
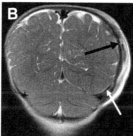
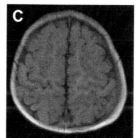
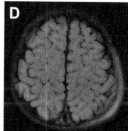

Fig. 5. Fast-brain MR imaging example using a fast head protocol in the acute setting in a child with left parietal fracture (*black arrow*), small subdural (*white arrow*), and scalp hematomas. (*A*) axial MPGR; (*B*) coronal SS FSE T2; (*C*) axial T1; and (*D*) axial FLAIR.

axial and sagittal T2 single-shot turbo spin echo, axial T1 turbo field echo, axial fluid-attenuated inversion recovery (FLAIR) single-shot turbo spin echo, axial gradient echo, and axial diffusion-weighted single-shot turbo spin echo planar imaging (Box 1), with all imaging obtained at a median imaging time of 365 seconds.[21]

Finally, with respect to abusive head trauma, ultrafast head MR has shown low sensitivity (50%–60%) for intracranial traumatic pathology, compared with NCCT or conventional MR imaging.[24]

Other investigators have highlighted that the use of MR imaging in the acute setting comes with important limitations. Studies using fast MR imaging have been performed in relatively stable patients, with limited data on the use of fast MR imaging for the acutely unstable patients, where immediate imaging findings guide management decisions. In addition, in many centers MR imaging and an immediate read of imaging is much less available after hours compared with CT.[25] MR imaging is inferior to CT for the detection of linear nondisplaced skull fractures.[21] A new technique called zero echo time (TE) skull imaging has shown some promise in the detection of skull fractures. In an article by Cho and colleagues,[26] zero TE imaging had diagnostic image quality comparable with CT; all skull fractures in the 13 patients included in their study could be seen on both MR imaging and CT.

2. Specific MR imaging sequences:
   a. *Susceptibility-weighted imaging (SWI)* (Figs. 4C, 8)SWI is a 3-dimensional (3D) gradient-echo MR sequence that gathers filtered-phase and magnitude data, allowing comparison of magnetic susceptibility differences among tissues.[27] SWI easily identifies the paramagnetic qualities of blood products, making this sequence more sensitive for detection of hemorrhagic traumatic brain lesions in children.[28,29] These findings might not be visible on T2*-weighted gradient echo sequences.[30] In a study by Beauchamp and colleagues,[31] the investigators compared the ability of CT versus MR imaging and SWI in detecting hemorrhagic lesions in 76 pediatric patients after TBI, with SWI performed about 5 weeks after injury, and found that SWI detected higher a number of hemorrhagic TBI than conventional MR imaging sequences and CT (86% vs 56% vs 68%, respectively). SWI is highly sensitive for visualization of DAI injury pattern, such as acute and early subacute microhemorrhages, which are used for prognostication in TBI.[32] For example, Tong and colleagues[33] found that the number and volume of hemorrhagic lesions detected with SWI correlates with long-term outcome using the Pediatric Cerebral Performance Scale. In their study, children with lower GCS scores (≤ 8, n = 30) or prolonged coma (>4 days, n = 20) had a greater average number ($p = 0.007$) and volume ($p = 0.008$) of hemorrhagic lesions. With respect to outcomes at 6 to 12 months after trauma, children with normal outcomes or mild disability (n = 30) had on average, less number ($p = 0.003$) and lower volume ($p = 0.003$) of hemorrhagic lesions, compared with those children who were moderately or severely disabled or in a vegetative state.[33] When comparing regional injury with clinical variables, the investigators also found significant differences in detecting hemorrhagic DAI when using SWI as compared with conventional T2*-weighted gradient-echo sequences, with higher sensitivity of SWI, allowing a more accurate and objective assessment of injury early after trauma and providing improved prognostic information on the duration of coma and long-term outcome.[33]

   b. *Diffusion-weighted imaging (DWI)* (Figs. 7, 9)—literature has shown that DWI can detect more DAI lesions within the first 48 hours of injury and identify additional shearing injuries that are not detected with T2-weighted fast spin-echo/FLAIR or GRE T2*-weighted sequence. However, DWI is less sensitive than T2* for hemorrhagic lesions detection.[34,35] Studies have shown that diffusion changes seen in white matter, which seem otherwise normal in patients who underwent

---

Box 1

Fast-brain MR imaging sequences

(3T preferable)

Suggested sequences as in article by Lindberg and colleagues (reference[21])

Axial single-shot TSE

Sagittal single-shot TSE

Axial T1 TFE

Axial FLAIR single-shot TSE

Axial gradient echo

Axial diffusion-weighted single-shot TSE planar imaging

Imaging obtained at a median imaging time of 365 seconds.

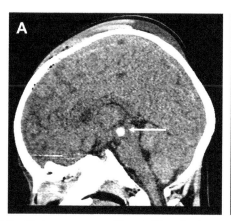
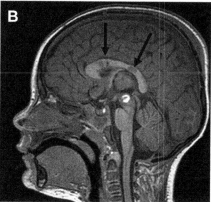

Fig. 6. (*A*) Sagittal non-contrast CT and (*B*) sagittal 3D-T1 MR imaging. CT shows a scalp hematoma and hyperdense mesencephalic hemorrhage (*white arrow*). MR imaging demonstrates hemorrhage in the brainstem (clarification of interpeduncular blood vs Duret hemorrhage, important for prognosis) and shear injuries corpus callosum (*black arrow*), the latter not seen with CT.

traumatic injury, differ from that seen in healthy controls brains, representing microstructural injury.[32] In a prospective study by Moen and colleagues,[32] they showed that the number of lesions detected with DWI in the corpus callosum and brainstem predicted outcome significantly and independently for patients with severe TBI, suggesting that DWI lesions may be due to a more extensive injury. DWI can also be useful for the diagnosis of fat embolism syndrome.[36]

c. FLAIR—FLAIR identifies non-hemorrhagic lesions such as edema (Fig. 1C) or gliosis in

the early and chronic phases, respectively, focal parenchymal lesions, contusions, lesions in the deep brain structures and brainstem, DAI, and subarachnoid hemorrhage.[32,37,38] It has shown higher sensitivity in detecting DAI, cortical contusions, and SDH and is superior to CT for detecting different TBI lesions due to the increased tissue contrast between grey and white matter by suppressing the fluid/CSF signal.[39] FLAIR has been used in patients during the first 4 weeks after severe TBI, estimating the volume of lesions in the corpus callosum,

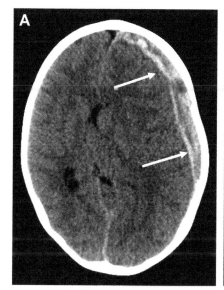
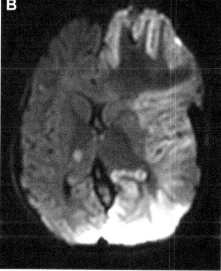

Fig. 7. (*A*) Axial non-contrast CT shows a large left frontoparietal subdural hemorrhage (*white arrows*) and possible early loss of grey-white matter differentiation, with mass effect and midline shift. After craniotomy, (*B*) axial DWI demonstrates extensive parenchymal ischemia with contralateral thalamic injury.

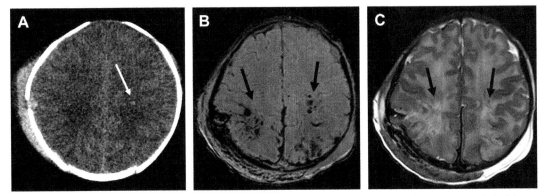

Fig. 8. (*A*) Axial non-contrast CT shows large right parietal bone fracture and right parieto-occipital hematoma. Beneath the fracture there is a small extra-axial hemorrhage and small hemorrhagic contusion. Few foci also seen in the left frontoparietal white matter (*white arrow*). (*B*) Axial SWI and (*C*) axial T2 demonstrate more extensive intraparenchymal hemorrhage in the right parietal lobe that is herniating through the fracture site, with blooming on SWI, multiple scattered punctate foci of SWI blooming in the bilateral frontoparietal lobes (*black arrows*), and a small right parietal subdural hemorrhage extending into the posterior interhemispheric region

brainstem, and thalamus, significantly improving the predicted outcome.[32,37,38] FLAIR, in combination with iron-sensitive sequences, is particularly useful in identifying DAI in locations such as the corpus callosum and fornix.[35] The early MR imaging, quantity and location of high signal intensity FLAIR lesions in pediatric patients after severe TBI have been used as a TBI imaging biomarker and demonstrated implications to predict long-term neurological outcome.[18]

CONVENTIONAL MR IMAGING PROTOCOL IN TRAUMATIC BRAIN INJURY

The standard conventional MR imaging protocol for TBI vary from site to site but includes at least a volumetric 3D T1, coronal T2 fast spin echo, and axial 2D FLAIR sequences, SWI and DWI.

In an article by Ferrazzano and colleagues, the investigators collected imaging practice information from 27 institutions; 67% of sites obtained T2*-weighted gradient recalled echo scans, 71% obtained SWI, with 80% of centers obtaining at least one of these sequences. Many sites (37%) reported that they performed both these sequences in severe TBI and 93% of sites included DWI. Other techniques such as perfusion-weighted imaging, DTI, or MR spectroscopy were performed much less frequently in TBI (29%, 39%, and 7%, respectively).[40] At the authors' institution, conventional MR imaging is defined in Box 2.

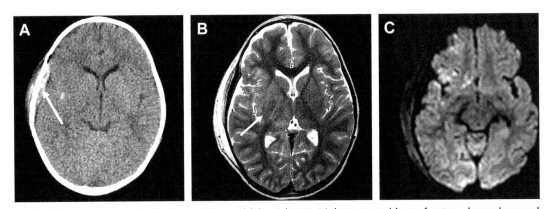

Fig. 9. (*A*) Axial non-contrast CT; (*B*) axial T2; and (*C*) axial DWI. Right temporal bone fracture, hyperdense subdural hematoma (*white arrow*), and right frontal contusion on non-contrast CT. MR imaging demonstrates extensive edema with foci of diffusion restriction in inferior right frontal and temporal lobes and right basal ganglia T2 hyperintensity (*white arrow*).

Box 2
Standard brain MR imaging sequences for pediatric traumatic brain injury

(3 T or 1.5 T)

Brain

    Sagittal T1 3D

    Axial 2D FLAIR

    Axial DWI (B1000)

    Axial SWI

    Coronal T2

Additional spine MR imaging sequences for trauma assessment

Cervical spine

    3 planes T2 FS

    Sagittal T1

    Axial 2 mm 0 gap mid-clivus to the C2/3 disc

    Sagittal T2 FS thoracolumbar spine

SUMMARY

Pediatric TBI is a worldwide issue. CT remains the mainstay for imaging in patients with acute TBI on a worldwide scale due to availability, ease of use, and speed. There is, however, a role for MR imaging both in the stable patient and with fast-brain imaging protocols both for the initial diagnosis and follow-up imaging. Advantages of MR imaging include superior soft tissue resolution and advanced ability to detect small hemorrhagic and nonhemorrhagic lesions that contribute to both diagnosis and prognostication. The ability to also reduce exposure to ionizing radiation in children is also a consideration.

CLINICS CARE POINTS

- The first line of imaging in pediatric head trauma is CT for rapidity, ease of use, and lack of need for sedation.

- MR imaging is helpful in the setting of a patient whose initial imaging is normal but neurological symptoms persist.

- MR imaging is warranted for prognosticating in severe TBI and to assess for locations of hemorrhages including brainstem hemorrhage.

- Fast MR imaging can be used to screen for injury in mild TBI but has a low sensitivity for fractures.

REFERENCES

1. Araki T, Yokota H, Morita A. Pediatric traumatic brain injury: characteristic features, diagnosis, and management. Neurol Med Chir (Tokyo) 2017;57(2):82–93.

2. Au AK, Clark RSB. Paediatric traumatic brain injury: prognostic insights and outlooks. Curr Opin Neurol 2017;30(6):565–72.

3. Kuppermann N, Holmes JF, Dayan PS, et al. Identification of children at very low risk of clinically-important brain injuries after head trauma: a prospective cohort study. Lancet 2009;374(9696):1160–70.

4. Hutchison JS, Emery C, Gagnon I, et al. The canadian traumatic brain injury research consortium: epitomizing collaborative research in canada. J Neurotrauma 2018;35(16):1858–63.

5. Roozenbeek B, Maas AI, Menon DK. Changing patterns in the epidemiology of traumatic brain injury. Nat Rev Neurol 2013;9(4):231–6.

6. Wintermark M, Coombs L, Druzgal TJ, et al. Traumatic brain injury imaging research roadmap. AJNR Am J Neuroradiol 2015;36(3):E12–23.

7. Bernardi B, Zimmerman RA, Bilaniuk LT. Neuroradiologic evaluation of pediatric craniocerebral trauma. Top Magn Reson Imaging 1993;5(3):161–73.

8. Gentry LR, Godersky JC, Thompson B, et al. Prospective comparative study of intermediate-field MR and CT in the evaluation of closed head trauma. AJR Am J Roentgenol 1988;150(3):673–82.

9. Pinto PS, Poretti A, Meoded A, et al. The unique features of traumatic brain injury in children. Review of the characteristics of the pediatric skull and brain, mechanisms of trauma, patterns of injury, complications and their imaging findings–part 1. J Neuroimaging 2012;22(2):e1–17.

10. Keenan HT, Runyan DK, Marshall SW, et al. A population-based study of inflicted traumatic brain injury in young children. JAMA 2003;290(5):621–6.

11. Ghajar J, Hariri RJ. Management of pediatric head injury. Pediatr Clin North Am 1992;39(5):1093–125.

12. Margulies SS, Thibault KL. Infant skull and suture properties: measurements and implications for mechanisms of pediatric brain injury. J Biomech Eng 2000;122(4):364–71.

13. Pinto PS, Meoded A, Poretti A, et al. The unique features of traumatic brain injury in children. review of the characteristics of the pediatric skull and brain, mechanisms of trauma, patterns of injury, complications, and their imaging findings–part 2. J Neuroimaging 2012;22(2):e18–41.

14. Expert Panel on Pediatric I, Ryan ME, Pruthi S, et al. ACR appropriateness criteria(R) head trauma-child. J Am Coll Radiol 2020;17(5S):S125–37.

15. Ryan ME, Palasis S, Saigal G, et al. ACR appropriateness criteria head trauma–child. J Am Coll Radiol 2014;11(10):939–47.

16. Servadei F, Nasi MT, Giuliani G, et al. CT prognostic factors in acute subdural haematomas: the value of the 'worst' CT scan. Br J Neurosurg 2000;14(2): 110–6.

17. Smith LGF, Milliron E, Ho ML, et al. Advanced neuroimaging in traumatic brain injury: an overview. Neurosurg Focus 2019;47(6):E17.

18. Smitherman E, Hernandez A, Stavinoha PL, et al. Predicting outcome after pediatric traumatic brain injury by early magnetic resonance imaging lesion location and volume. J Neurotrauma 2016;33(1): 35–48.

19. Hesselink JR, Dowd CF, Healy ME, et al. MR imaging of brain contusions: a comparative study with CT. AJR Am J Roentgenol 1988;150(5):1133–42.

20. Kara A, Celik SE, Dalbayrak S, et al. Magnetic resonance imaging finding in severe head injury patients with normal computerized tomography. Turk Neurosurg 2008;18(1):1–9.

21. Lindberg DM, Stence NV, Grubenhoff JA, et al. Feasibility and accuracy of fast MRI versus CT for traumatic brain injury in young children. Pediatrics 2019;144(4). https://doi.org/10.1542/peds.2019-0419.

22. Mehta H, Acharya J, Mohan AL, et al. Minimizing radiation exposure in evaluation of pediatric head trauma: use of rapid MR imaging. AJNR Am J Neuroradiol 2016;37(1):11–8.

23. Young JY, Duhaime AC, Caruso PA, et al. Comparison of non-sedated brain MRI and CT for the detection of acute traumatic injury in children 6 years of age or less. Emerg Radiol 2016;23(4):325–31.

24. Kralik SF, Yasrebi M, Supakul N, et al. Diagnostic performance of ultrafast brain MRI for evaluation of abusive head trauma. AJNR Am J Neuroradiol 2017;38(4):807–13.

25. Burstein B, Saint-Martin C. The feasibility of fast MRI to reduce CT radiation exposure with acute traumatic head injuries. Pediatrics 2019;144(4). https://doi.org/10.1542/peds.2019-2387.

26. Cho SB, Baek HJ, Ryu KH, et al. Clinical feasibility of Zero TE Skull MRI in patients with head trauma in comparison with CT: a single-center study. AJNR Am J Neuroradiol 2019;40(1):109–15.

27. Mittal S, Wu Z, Neelavalli J, et al. Susceptibility-weighted imaging: technical aspects and clinical applications, part 2. AJNR Am J Neuroradiol 2009; 30(2):232–52.

28. Barlow KM. Traumatic brain injury. Handb Clin Neurol 2013;112:891–904.

29. Haacke EM, Xu Y, Cheng YC, et al. Susceptibility weighted imaging (SWI). Magn Reson Med 2004; 52(3):612–8.

30. Tong KA, Ashwal S, Holshouser BA, et al. Hemorrhagic shearing lesions in children and adolescents with posttraumatic diffuse axonal injury: improved detection and initial results. Radiology 2003;227(2): 332–9.

31. Beauchamp MH, Ditchfield M, Babl FE, et al. Detecting traumatic brain lesions in children: CT versus MRI versus susceptibility weighted imaging (SWI). J Neurotrauma 2011;28(6):915–27.

32. Moen KG, Brezova V, Skandsen T, et al. Traumatic axonal injury: the prognostic value of lesion load in corpus callosum, brain stem, and thalamus in different magnetic resonance imaging sequences. J Neurotrauma 2014;31(17):1486–96.

33. Tong KA, Ashwal S, Holshouser BA, et al. Diffuse axonal injury in children: clinical correlation with hemorrhagic lesions. Ann Neurol 2004;56(1):36–50.

34. Huisman TA, Sorensen AG, Hergan K, et al. Diffusion-weighted imaging for the evaluation of diffuse axonal injury in closed head injury. J Comput Assist Tomogr 2003;27(1):5–11.

35. Le TH, Gean AD. Neuroimaging of traumatic brain injury. Mt Sinai J Med 2009;76(2):145–62.

36. Ryu CW, Lee DH, Kim TK, et al. Cerebral fat embolism: diffusion-weighted magnetic resonance imaging findings. Acta Radiol 2005;46(5):528–33.

37. Mittl RL, Grossman RI, Hiehle JF, et al. Prevalence of MR evidence of diffuse axonal injury in patients with mild head injury and normal head CT findings. AJNR Am J Neuroradiol 1994;15(8):1583–9.

38. Singer MB, Atlas SW, Drayer BP. Subarachnoid space disease: diagnosis with fluid-attenuated inversion-recovery MR imaging and comparison with gadolinium-enhanced spin-echo MR imaging–blinded reader study. Radiology 1998;208(2): 417–22.

39. Ashikaga R, Araki Y, Ishida O. MRI of head injury using FLAIR. Neuroradiology 1997;39(4):239–42.

40. Ferrazzano PA, Rosario BL, Wisniewski SR, et al. Use of magnetic resonance imaging in severe pediatric traumatic brain injury: assessment of current practice. J Neurosurg Pediatr 2019;23(4):471–9.

Imaging Approach to Concussion

Jeffrey B. Ware, MD[a],*, Danielle K. Sandsmark, MD, PhD[b]

KEYWORDS

- Concussion • mTBI • CTE • Subconcussion • MR imaging

KEY POINTS

- Insights from neuroimaging research over the past few decades are changing the conception of mild traumatic brain injury (mTBI) from a static, self-limited, and primarily functional disturbance to a pathophysiological process that evolves over time.
- Research increasingly ties chronic post-concussive symptoms and cognitive difficulties to microstructural and physiological disturbances in the brain.
- Owing to the complex and multifaceted nature of TBI pathophysiology a wide range of imaging techniques is necessary to comprehensively assess the neurobiological manifestations.
- Abnormalities in advanced MR imaging biomarkers of mTBI often persist beyond the point of clinical recovery from concussion, raising the question of whether the period of heightened vulnerability to repeat injury is longer than previously recognized.
- Advanced MR imaging techniques capable of detecting microstructural and microvascular injuries occult on conventional MR imaging remain primarily in the research realm; however, with additional research geared towards reliable individual-level assessment, clinical translation may be on the horizon.

INTRODUCTION

Once considered a self-limited and primarily functional disturbance, the acute and long-term neurobiological sequelae of concussion (also referred to as mild traumatic brain injury, or mTBI) and subconcussive head trauma have become increasingly evident in recent decades owing to several lines of research including neuroimaging. Whereas the acute neurological dysfunction associated with mTBI most commonly resolves over the first several days to weeks after injury, it is now well-recognized that post-concussive symptoms and cognitive deficits may become chronic within a sizable subset of patients. Furthermore, associations between neuropathological changes of chronic traumatic encephalopathy (CTE) and repetitive mild head trauma, along with strengthened epidemiological links between TBI and neurodegenerative disease later in life, particularly among populations vulnerable to repeat trauma have brought tremendous public attention to the long-term implications of these injuries.

Neuroimaging, although traditionally used in the clinical management of mTBI for the identification of intracranial lesions warranting urgent neurosurgical intervention, changes in medical management, or close monitoring is increasingly employed for the detection of less-severe post-traumatic brain lesions, which may carry important prognostic significance. Furthermore, the use of advanced, quantitative MR imaging techniques in research settings has led to several important insights on the pathophysiology of mTBI, ultimately converging upon the notion that negative clinical neuroimaging findings in TBI owe more to the limited sensitivity of current clinical imaging techniques than to the absence of neuropathology. Microstructural and physiological derangements associated with mTBI are detectable with

[a] Department of Radiology, Neuroradiology Division, University of Pennsylvania, 3400 Spruce Street, Philadelphia, PA 19104, USA; [b] Department of Neurology, University of Pennsylvania, 3400 Spruce Street, Philadelphia, PA 19104, USA
* Corresponding author.
E-mail address: Jeffrey.Ware2@pennmedicine.upenn.edu

Neuroimag Clin N Am 33 (2023) 261–269
https://doi.org/10.1016/j.nic.2023.01.002
1052-5149/23/

advanced MR imaging techniques and have been increasingly linked to prolonged recovery and the development of persistent post-concussive symptoms across the spectrum of clinical severity. Research on imaging biomarkers of mTBI suggests that neurobiological derangements may, at least in some cases, persist beyond the point of clinical recovery, and furthermore may even occur in the absence of immediate clinical manifestations. These insights are helping to shift the conceptualization of TBI from a single injury event to a pathophysiological process that evolves over time, and ultimately provide a strong rationale for pursuing clinical translation of advanced neuroimaging to monitor these changes more directly in individual patients.

CLINICAL PROBLEM

TBI is typically classified as mild based on the initial Glasgow Coma Scale (GCS) of 13 to 15, no or brief (<30 min) loss of consciousness, and a duration of post-traumatic amnesia of less than 24 h. mTBI accounts for approximately 80% of all TBI in the United States, and therefore, the vast majority of the estimated 2.8 million TBI-related emergency department visits per year.[1] The incidence of mTBI has risen in recent decades,[2] and is likely to be underestimated as in many cases no medical care is sought. The totality of economic and social burden resulting from mTBI given such high incidence and prevalence is considerable, and only magnified with increasing use of more sensitive assessments better suited for the detection of more subtle cognitive and behavioral effects of milder TBIs,[3] as well as effects manifesting years after injury.[4] Although the acute deterioration of mTBI patients is rare,[5] post-concussive symptoms such as headaches, irritability, dizziness, sleep disturbances, light and noise sensitivity, as well as deficits in memory, concentration, and other cognitive functions are commonly present in the days to weeks after mTBI.[6] These symptoms are expected to resolve by 3 months in the majority of patients; however, persistent post-concussive symptoms are observed in as many as 41% at 6 months post-injury,[7] with up to 30% developing a new or worsening post-concussive symptom 3 months after injury. mTBI patients with a pre-injury neuropsychiatric disorder appear to be at the highest risk of the development of post-concussive symptoms.[8] The primary goal of clinical management after excluding emergent and alternative etiologies is to prevent the persistence of these symptoms. Recently, more proactive and graded approaches are increasingly favored in lieu of traditional prolonged rest in light of recent evidence for the effectiveness of early interventions such as early graded aerobic exercise in reducing symptom burden and persistence.[9] Although return-to-activity decisions have typically been based on the resolution of clinical symptoms, evidence for the persistence of disturbances in brain metabolism, cerebrovascular function, and network connectivity beyond the resolution of post-concussive symptoms suggests that physiologic recovery from brain injury occurs within a longer timeframe than clinical recovery,[10] and question whether the period of vulnerability to repeat injury may be greater than previously recognized.

In addition to the development and persistence of post-concussive symptoms and cognitive difficulties in the weeks to months after injury, there is increasing concern over the longer-term consequences of mTBI. Although moderate and severe TBI has long been considered a risk factor for developing late-life neurodegenerative diseases such as Alzheimer's disease, Parkinson's disease, and frontotemporal dementias,[11,12] recent evidence suggests this risk may also extend to those exposed to repetitive mTBIs and sub-concussive head trauma,[13] occurring over a prolonged latent period of several years to decades. The mechanisms which account for the development of trauma-related neurodegeneration (TReND)[12] are incompletely understood; however, the neuropathological changes of CTE, which have been identified among athletes, military veterans, and other individuals exposed to high levels of repetitive mild head trauma,[14] appear to be very rare among individuals without such history.[15] This suggests that although the clinical features may overlap with those of other neurogenerative conditions, neurodegeneration after TBI is a pathologically distinct process.

PATHOPHYSIOLOGY

The pathophysiology of TBI, which underlies the range of post-concussive symptomatology, cognitive dysfunction, and neurological deterioration, is complex and multifaceted, often referred to as a "neurometabolic cascade."[16] Linear and particularly rotational forces stemming from the initial impact result in stretching and/or disruption of axonal cell membranes,[17] which may lead to cell death or reactive changes without death.[18] Although complete axonal severance is rare in mTBI, axonal deformation and cytoskeletal disruption impair the process of axonal transport and therefore, neurotransmission, resulting in functional disconnection which may occur in the absence of neuronal cell death, recognizable pathologically as axonal swellings or varicosities.[19] Furthermore, force-induced mechanoporation can precipitate ionic flux and membrane depolarization,[16] producing indiscriminate release of glutamate leading to excitotoxicity. To restore ionic balance, ion pump use, and deplete cellular energy stores, creating a mismatch between energy demand and supply, especially when blood flow is compromised due to concomitant microvascular injury. The resultant metabolic dysfunction and associated altered glucose metabolism is also thought to underlie the period of heightened vulnerability to a second insult after mTBI.[20,21] Calcium influx driven by membrane depolarization further impairs metabolism, and promotes cytoskeletal phosphorylation and proteolytic damage along with the release of free radicals, which ultimately potentiates the loss of structural integrity and other forms of cellular damage while stimulating a neuroinflammatory response through the activation of quiescent microglia, release of cytokines, and resultant activation of immune cells. Neuroinflammation, which has been detected pathologically several years after a single TBI,[22] may represent a critical mechanism of neurodegeneration in the chronic phase of TBI.

Microvascular injuries occur alongside axonal shear injuries,[23–27] leading to dysfunction of the neurovascular unit (NVU) compromising cerebrovascular reactivity (CVR) and blood–brain barrier (BBB) integrity. NVU dysfunction impairs neural repair mechanisms and precipitates further brain tissue injury through a range of secondary pathological processes including chronic hypoperfusion, mitochondrial dysfunction, calcium dysregulation, neuroinflammation, and ultimately deposition of tau and amyloid.[28–31] The interaction between axonal injury and NVU dysfunction is postulated to initiate a feed-forward loop that eventually leads to the development TReND pathology, driving cognitive impairment.[12,32,33] Furthermore, as NVU dysfunction is increasingly implicated in the pathogenesis of other Alzheimer's disease-related dementias (ADRDs) including AD,[32,34] small vessel ischemic disease,[35] and frontotemporal lobar degeneration (FTLD)[36]; this may reflect a mechanism by which TBI may increase the risk for these neurodegenerative conditions.

The pathological hallmark and pathognomonic finding of CTE is the deposition of phosphorylated tau within neurons and astroglia distributed around small blood vessels in an irregular pattern at the depths of cortical sulci.[37] There are several additional supportive, though less specific, pathological features including TDP-43 pathology, reactive microgliosis, as well as midline abnormalities including enlargement of the 3rd ventricle, cavum septum pellucidum (CSP) and other septal abnormalities, atrophy of the mammillary bodies, hypothalamus, and corpus callosum.[37,38] Tau deposition in CTE stems from the microtubule disruption occurring with the initial axonal injury, with subsequent phosphorylation driving further misfolding and aggregation, and possibly even prion-like propagation. The stage of CTE pathology among a series of professional soccer players shows a stronger correlation with years of play as opposed to the number of concussions, suggesting that the primary driver of this process is repetitive mostly sub-concussive blows.[14]

IMAGING APPROACH

Although the diagnosis and stratification of TBI remain clinical based on appropriate history and measures such as the GCS and the duration of post-traumatic amnesia, neuroimaging plays an important role in guiding management. In the acute setting, the goal of clinical assessment is to identify patients at risk for serious damage and deterioration, which may be due to an expanding intracranial hematoma or progressive cerebral edema. In acute mTBI, computed tomography (CT) remains the first line imaging test for those patients in whom there is clinical suspicion for intra- or extra-axial hemorrhage, contusions, or skull fractures warranting urgent neurosurgical intervention, changes in medical management, or intensive monitoring.[39] Repeat head CT does not alter acute management when performed in patients without neurological decline.[40] MR imaging, which confers greater sensitivity for several traumatic lesions such as axonal injury, small hemorrhages, contusions, and small extra-axial collections[41,42] is typically reserved for those with neurological deficits out of proportion to findings on CT,[43] despite a relatively high positivity rate of approximately 30% in mTBI patients with normal head CT.[44,45] The presence of TBI-related intracranial lesions on both CT and MR imaging is associated with high rates of depressive and anxiety disorders, incomplete recovery, and other unfavorable outcomes.[44,46–48]

Conventional neuroimaging in the subacute and chronic post-injury periods has typically been used to rule out delayed structural (ie, subdural hematoma) and alternative neurological etiologies in patients with persistent post-concussive symptoms. As the gross pathological features of CTE and TReND are increasingly characterized; however, there is also motivation to examine the ability of conventional MR imaging to detect these features in vivo among individuals at risk (Fig. 1). A

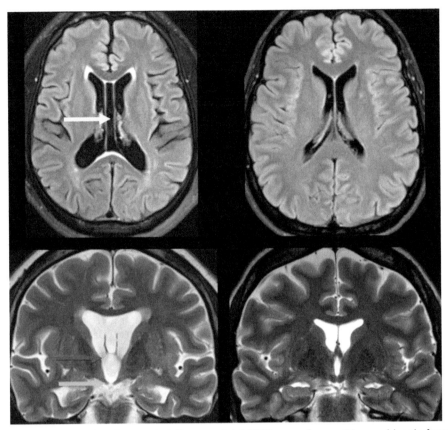

Fig. 1. Axial FLAIR (*top right*) and coronal T2 (*bottom right*) MRI images from a 45-year-old male former professional boxer who presented with cognitive impairment with comparable images from a healthy individual of similar age (*left*). The MR imaging shows diffuse brain atrophy with enlargement of the lateral and third ventricles, a large cavum septum pellucidum (*yellow arrow*), and striking atrophy of the fornices (*red arrow*) and mammillary bodies (*blue arrow*).

retrospective review of antemortem MR imaging examinations from pathologically confirmed cases of CTE showed radiologically detectable anterior frontotemporal atrophy patterns, larger lateral and third ventricles, higher incidence of a CSP.[49] Previous work has also shown higher incidence and size of CSP in those with a history of TBI or exposure to repetitive head trauma, with a direct correlation between CSP size and cognitive impairment[50]; the clinical utility of these features assessed at the individual level is limited, however, due to the poor specificity of findings such as CSP, which are present in a high proportion of healthy individuals,[51] and the poor sensitivity for identification of TBI-related neuropathology particularly early in the disease process when interventions would be expected to have the greatest likelihood of success. Recent work showing the limited utility of neuroradiological MR imaging evaluation for detecting a range of TBI–related abnormalities in high-contact sports athletes further underscores the need for more sensitive approaches.[52]

ADVANCED MR IMAGING IN MILD TRAUMATIC BRAIN INJURY AND SUB-CONCUSSION

The conception of mTBI in the context of normal conventional neuroimaging as a solely functional injury has largely been abandoned in large part due to a body of research accumulated over the past few decades applying a range of high-sensitivity advanced MR imaging techniques to mTBI and sub-concussive head trauma. Owing to the complexity of TBI pathophysiology, a range of neuroimaging techniques are necessary to fully assess the biological manifestations. These include methods to quantitatively measure microstructural and microvascular damage, which are below the resolution of qualitative neuroradiological assessment, as well as methods for assessing brain physiology inaccessible using conventional MR imaging sequences, many of which are reviewed in greater detail elsewhere in this collection. Generally, research employing these techniques increasingly suggests that adverse pathological changes occur in the brain after mTBI and in association with repetitive sub-concussive head trauma.

Microstructural injuries associated with mTBI have been studied most extensively using diffusion MR imaging techniques such as diffusion tensor imaging (DTI), which exploits water diffusion-sensitive sequences to draw inferences on the organization of white matter fibers and other microstructural properties. A wealth of DTI studies over the past 15 years have consistently suggested that axonal pathology is occurring after mTBI even when conventional brain MR imaging sequences are normal, with DTI parameter alterations most frequently observed in large white matter bundles such as the corpus callosum, internal capsule, and long association pathways.[53] This notion is also supported by histopathological studies of showing the presence of diffuse axonal injury in patients with mild TBI who died from other injuries sustained concurrently.[54] The most common pattern of DTI alteration particularly in the subacute to chronic phase of adult mTBI is reduced fractional anisotropy (FA) and elevated mean diffusivity (MD),[53] believed based on DTI studies in animal models to reflect axonal injury, Wallerian degeneration, demyelination, and/or edema.[55] DTI findings in mTBI, however, have not been entirely consistent with some studies suggesting the reverse pattern of elevated FA and MD, particularly in studies of acute and pediatric mTBI.[53] DTI injury burden tends to correlate with cognitive deficits[56] and other outcomes,[57] adding to outcome prediction over MR imaging alone.[58] Interestingly, exposure to sub-concussive head impacts has also been shown to correlate negatively with changes in white matter FA over the course of a high school football season.[59]

Microvascular injury is a frequent pathological manifestation of TBI across the spectrum of injury severities.[23-27] Cerebral microhemorrhages, for which susceptibility-weighted imaging (SWI) is more sensitive than CT and conventional MR imaging sequences,[60] are indicative of traumatic microvascular injury, particularly when in a linear configuration[61,62] or clustered in a particular distribution such as along the grey-white junction, corpus callosum, or brainstem. Microhemorrhages have been reported in up to 30% of patients with mTBI,[44] and have generally been correlated with injury severity[60,63] and poor outcomes.[64] The prevalence is likely to be much lower, however, among mTBI patients who do not seek emergency room care as well as in association with sub-concussive head trauma.[65,66] Perfusion imaging techniques such as arterial spin labeling (ASL) have also been used to assess microvascular function in mTBI, and generally suggest that alterations in cerebral blood flow (CBF) are associated with mTBI, with most studies suggesting a reduction in CBF and a minority of studies finding an increase.[67] Though a few studies have identified a correlation between CBF alterations and post-concussive symptoms[68] as well as cognitive performance,[69] a consistent relationship with clinical symptoms has not emerged.[67] Inconsistent findings between studies may relate to differences in timing of assessment as longitudinal studies suggest decreases in CBF over the post-mTBI recovery period, which interestingly appears persistently abnormal beyond the point of symptom resolution.[70] ASL perfusion is also limited, however, by the inability to disentangle primary microvascular injury from perfusion changes secondary to metabolic derangements, which are likely to occur in mTBI. A more specific measure of microvascular function that has been assessed in mTBI is CVR, or the normal vasodilatory response of cerebral arterioles to vasomotor stimuli, which can be quantified by measuring the blood oxygen level-dependent (BOLD) MR imaging signal response to hypercapnia. CVR deficits, which have been shown in association with mTBI,[71,72] reflect an inability of the microvasculature to regulate tissue blood supply in accordance with metabolic demand, which in turn can potentiate neuronal damage and dysfunction.

Brain tissue loss reflecting the cumulative effect of these pathological processes and which is often below the resolution of routine radiological assessment is detectable over the course of months to years after mTBI using quantitative measures of cortical thickness, subcortical grey, and white matter volumes, as well as CSF space volumes computationally extracted from high-resolution T1-weighted images.[73-76] Subtle but statistically significant brain volume loss has also been observed among those participating in contact sports without having sustained mTBI.[65,75] The distribution of atrophy across studies has been variable; however cortical thinning is most frequently observed in a frontotemporal pattern including the hippocampus and amygdala, and subcortical-volume loss commonly involves structures near the midline such as the upper brainstem, thalamus, corpus callosum, and cingulum.[77] Although a particular pattern of atrophy specific to TBI has yet to clearly emerge, there is some evidence that a more specific feature of TBI-related atrophy is disproportionate cortical volume loss along sulci relative to gyri owing to disproportionate distribution of shearing forces during trauma.[78]

SUMMARY

Neuroimaging has played a major role in advancing the understanding of mTBI pathophysiology and in revealing the associated microstructural and microvascular injuries in vivo. Insights gained over the past two decades of imaging research are helping to drive a shift in the conceptualization of TBI from a single injury event to a pathophysiological process that evolves over time and may even occur in the absence of overt clinical manifestations. Although the role of neuroimaging in the acute and long-term clinical care of patients with mTBI is established, there remains a great yet largely unfilled potential for the clinical translation of advanced MR imaging techniques to detect and monitor the biological manifestations of mTBI in individual patients. Additional efforts geared toward standardizing data collection and analysis procedures, harmonization, and data aggregation to establish normative references that will be essential for clinical translation and reliable assessments of individual patients. The promise of more accurate prediction of clinical course, identification of brain injury endophenotypes, and monitoring of recovery and therapeutic efficacy provides strong motivation to continue these efforts.

CLINICS CARE POINTS

- Computed tomography has an established role in the acute clinical management of mild traumatic brain injury for detecting intracranial lesions warranting urgent interventions.

- Recognition of the prognostic significance of traumatic intracranial lesions is motivating the wider use of MR imaging for detecting traumatic intracranial sequelae in the acute to subacute post-injury time period.

- Although some macroscopic features of chronic traumatic encephalopathy (CTE) are detectable with MR imaging, these features lack specificity, and there is a great need to develop imaging biomarkers of CTE and associated chronic TBI pathology.

- Advanced MR imaging techniques capable of detecting microstructural and microvascular injuries occult on conventional MR imaging remain primarily in the research realm; however, with additional research geared toward reliable individual-level assessment clinical translation may be on the horizon.

DISCLOSURE

The authors have nothing to disclose.

ACKNOWLEDGMENT

We acknowledge the following reasearch grant (PI Ware) R01 NS125408/NS/NINDS NIH HHS/United States.

REFERENCES

1. Taylor CA, Bell JM, Breiding MJ, et al. Traumatic brain injury-related emergency department visits, hospitalizations, and deaths - United States, 2007 and 2013. MMWR Surveill Summ 2017;66(9):1–16.
2. Marin JR, Weaver MD, Yealy DM, et al. Trends in visits for traumatic brain injury to emergency departments in the United States. JAMA 2014;311(18):1917.
3. Narayan RK, Michel ME, Ansell B, et al. Clinical trials in head injury. J Neurotrauma 2002;19(5):503–57.
4. McKinlay A, Grace R, Horwood J, et al. Adolescent psychiatric symptoms following preschool childhood mild traumatic brain injury: evidence from a birth cohort. J Head Trauma Rehabil 2009;24(3):221–7.
5. Chojak R, Koźba-Gosztyła M, Pawłowski M, et al. Deterioration after mild traumatic brain injury: a single-center experience with cost analysis. Front Neurol 2021;12:588429.
6. Carroll LJ, Cassidy JD, Peloso PM, et al. Prognosis for mild traumatic brain injury: results of the WHO Collaborating Centre Task Force on Mild Traumatic Brain Injury. J Rehabil Med 2004;43(Suppl):84–105.
7. Cnossen MC, van der Naalt J, Spikman JM, et al. Prediction of persistent post-concussion symptoms after mild traumatic brain injury. J Neurotrauma 2018;35(22):2691–8.
8. Meares S, Shores EA, Taylor AJ, et al. The prospective course of postconcussion syndrome: the role of mild traumatic brain injury. Neuropsychology 2011;25(4):454–65.
9. Silverberg ND, Iaccarino MA, Panenka WJ, et al. Management of concussion and mild traumatic brain injury: a synthesis of practice guidelines. Arch Phys Med Rehabil 2020;101(2):382–93.
10. Kamins J, Bigler E, Covassin T, et al. What is the physiological time to recovery after concussion? A systematic review. Br J Sports Med 2017;51(12):935–40.
11. Zlokovic BV. Neurovascular pathways to neurodegeneration in Alzheimer's disease and other disorders. Nat Rev Neurosci 2011;12(12):723–38.
12. Smith DH, Johnson VE, Trojanowski JQ, et al. Chronic traumatic encephalopathy — confusion and controversies. Nat Rev Neurol 2019;15(3):179–83.

13. Mackay DF, Russell ER, Stewart K, et al. Neurodegenerative disease mortality among former professional soccer players. N Engl J Med 2019;381(19):1801–8.

14. McKee AC, Stern RA, Nowinski CJ, et al. The spectrum of disease in chronic traumatic encephalopathy. Brain 2013;136(Pt 1):43–64.

15. Bieniek KF, Ross OA, Cormier KA, et al. Chronic traumatic encephalopathy pathology in a neurodegenerative disorders brain bank. Acta Neuropathol 2015;130(6):877–89.

16. Giza CC, Hovda DA. The new neurometabolic cascade of concussion. Neurosurgery 2014;75(Suppl 4):S24–33.

17. Rowson S, Bland ML, Campolettano ET, et al. Biomechanical perspectives on concussion in sport. Sports Med Arthrosc Rev 2016;24(3):100–7.

18. Farkas O. Mechanoporation induced by diffuse traumatic brain injury: an irreversible or reversible response to injury? J Neurosci 2006;26(12):3130–40.

19. Johnson VE, Stewart W, Smith DH. Axonal pathology in traumatic brain injury. Exp Neurol 2013;246:35–43.

20. Prins ML, Alexander D, Giza CC, et al. Repeated mild traumatic brain injury: mechanisms of cerebral vulnerability. J Neurotrauma 2013;30(1):30–8.

21. Bergsneider M, Hovda DA, Lee SM, et al. Dissociation of cerebral glucose metabolism and level of consciousness during the period of metabolic depression following human traumatic brain injury. J Neurotrauma 2000;17(5):389–401.

22. Johnson VE, Stewart JE, Begbie FD, et al. Inflammation and white matter degeneration persist for years after a single traumatic brain injury. Brain 2013;136(1):28–42.

23. DeWitt DS, Prough DS. Traumatic cerebral vascular injury: the effects of concussive brain injury on the cerebral vasculature. J Neurotrauma 2003;20(9):795–825.

24. Kenney K, Amyot F, Haber M, et al. Cerebral vascular injury in traumatic brain injury. Exp Neurol 2016;275:353–66.

25. Castejón OJ. Ultrastructural pathology of cortical capillary pericytes in human traumatic brain oedema. Folia Neuropathol 2011;49(3):162–73.

26. Castejón OJ. Ultrastructural alterations of human cortical capillary basement membrane in human brain oedema. Folia Neuropathol 2014;52(1):10–21.

27. Sandsmark DK, Bashir A, Wellington CL, et al. Cerebral microvascular injury: a potentially treatable endophenotype of traumatic brain injury-induced neurodegeneration. Neuron 2019;103(3):367–79.

28. Golding EM, Robertson CS, Bryan RM. The consequences of traumatic brain injury on cerebral blood flow and autoregulation: a review. Clin Exp Hypertens 1999;21(4):299–332.

29. Golding E. Sequelae following traumatic brain injury The cerebrovascular perspective. Brain Res Rev 2002;38(3):377–88.

30. Szarka N, Pabbidi MR, Amrein K, et al. Traumatic Brain Injury Impairs Myogenic Constriction of Cerebral Arteries: Role of Mitochondria-Derived H2O2 and TRPV4-Dependent Activation of BKca Channels. J Neurotrauma 2018. https://doi.org/10.1089/neu.2017.5056.

31. Kisler K, Nelson AR, Rege SV, et al. Pericyte degeneration leads to neurovascular uncoupling and limits oxygen supply to brain. Nat Neurosci 2017;20(3):406–16.

32. Ramos-Cejudo J, Wisniewski T, Marmar C, et al. Traumatic brain injury and Alzheimer's disease: the cerebrovascular link. EBioMedicine 2018;28:21–30.

33. Iadecola C. The neurovascular unit coming of age: a journey through neurovascular coupling in health and disease. Neuron 2017;96(1):17–42.

34. Sweeney MD, Kisler K, Montagne A, et al. The role of brain vasculature in neurodegenerative disorders. Nat Neurosci 2018;21(10):1318–31.

35. Sam K, Conklin J, Holmes KR, et al. Impaired dynamic cerebrovascular response to hypercapnia predicts development of white matter hyperintensities. NeuroImage: Clin 2016;11:796–801.

36. Olm CA, Kandel BM, Avants BB, et al. Arterial spin labeling perfusion predicts longitudinal decline in semantic variant primary progressive aphasia. J Neurol 2016;263(10):1927–38.

37. Bieniek KF, Cairns NJ, Crary JF, et al. The second NINDS/NIBIB consensus meeting to define neuropathological criteria for the diagnosis of chronic traumatic encephalopathy. J Neuropathol Exp Neurol 2021;80(3):210–9.

38. McKee AC, Cairns NJ, Dickson DW, et al. The first NINDS/NIBIB consensus meeting to define neuropathological criteria for the diagnosis of chronic traumatic encephalopathy. Acta Neuropathol 2016;131(1):75–86.

39. Expert Panel on Neurological Imaging, Shih RY, Burns J, et al. ACR appropriateness criteria® head trauma: 2021 update. J Am Coll Radiol 2021;18(5S):S13–36.

40. Sifri ZC, Homnick AT, Vaynman A, et al. a prospective evaluation of the value of repeat cranial computed tomography in patients with minimal head injury and an intracranial bleed. J Trauma Inj Infect Crit Care 2006;61(4):862–7.

41. Gentry L, Godersky J, Thompson B. MR imaging of head trauma: review of the distribution and radiopathologic features of traumatic lesions. Am J Roentgenology 1988;150(3):663–72.

42. Hesselink, Dowd C, Healy M, et al. MR imaging of brain contusions: a comparative study with CT. Am J Roentgenology 1988;150(5):1133–42.

43. Wintermark M, Sanelli PC, Anzai Y, et al, on behalf of the American College of Radiology Head Injury Institute. Imaging evidence and recommendations for traumatic brain injury: advanced neuro- and neurovascular imaging techniques. Am J Neuroradiology 2015;36(2):E1–11.

44. Yuh EL, Mukherjee P, Lingsma HF, et al. Magnetic resonance imaging improves 3-month outcome prediction in mild traumatic brain injury: MRI in MTBI. Ann Neurol 2013;73(2):224–35.

45. Yue JK, Yuh EL, Korley FK, et al. Association between plasma GFAP concentrations and MRI abnormalities in patients with CT-negative traumatic brain injury in the TRACK-TBI cohort: a prospective multicentre study. Lancet Neurol 2019;18(10): 953–61.

46. Yuh EL, Jain S, Sun X, et al. Pathological computed tomography features associated with adverse outcomes after mild traumatic brain injury: a TRACK-TBI study with external validation in CENTER-TBI. JAMA Neurol 2021;78(9):1137.

47. Sadowski-Cron C, Schneider J, Senn P, et al. Patients with mild traumatic brain injury: immediate and long-term outcome compared to intra-cranial injuries on CT scan. Brain Inj 2006;20(11):1131–7.

48. Bombardier CH. Rates of major depressive disorder and clinical outcomes following traumatic brain injury. JAMA 2010;303(19):1938.

49. Alosco ML, Mian AZ, Buch K, et al. Structural MRI profiles and tau correlates of atrophy in autopsy-confirmed CTE. Alz Res Ther 2021;13(1):193.

50. Lee JK, Wu J, Bullen J, et al. Association of cavum septum pellucidum and cavum vergae with cognition, mood, and brain volumes in professional fighters. JAMA Neurol 2020;77(1):35.

51. Das J M, Dossani RH. Cavum septum pellucidum. In: StatPearls. StatPearls Publishing; 2022. Available at: http://www.ncbi.nlm.nih.gov/books/NBK537048/. Accessed September 2, 2022.

52. McAllister D, Akers C, Boldt B, et al. Neuroradiologic evaluation of MRI in high-contact sports. Front Neurol 2021;12:701948.

53. Lindsey HM, Hodges CB, Greer KM, et al. Diffusion-weighted imaging in mild traumatic brain injury: a systematic review of the literature. Neuropsychol Rev 2021. https://doi.org/10.1007/s11065-021-09485-5.

54. Clark JM. Distribution of microglial clusters in the brain after head injury. J Neurol Neurosurg Psychiatry 1974;37(4):463–74.

55. Mac Donald CL, Dikranian K, Bayly P, et al. Diffusion tensor imaging reliably detects experimental traumatic axonal injury and indicates approximate time of injury. J Neurosci 2007;27(44):11869–76.

56. Niogi SN, Mukherjee P, Ghajar J, et al. Extent of microstructural white matter injury in postconcussive syndrome correlates with impaired cognitive reaction time: a 3T diffusion tensor imaging study of mild traumatic brain injury. Am J Neuroradiology 2008;29(5):967–73.

57. Schaefer PW, Huisman TAGM, Sorensen AG, et al. Diffusion-weighted MR imaging in closed head injury: high correlation with initial glasgow coma scale score and score on modified Rankin scale at discharge. Radiology 2004;233(1):58–66.

58. Richter S, Winzeck S, Kornaropoulos EN, et al. Neuroanatomical substrates and symptoms associated with magnetic resonance imaging of patients with mild traumatic brain injury. JAMA Netw Open 2021;4(3):e210994.

59. Bahrami N, Sharma D, Rosenthal S, et al. Subconcussive head impact exposure and white matter tract changes over a single season of youth football. Radiology 2016;281(3):919–26.

60. Tao JJ, Zhang WJ, Wang D, et al. Susceptibility weighted imaging in the evaluation of hemorrhagic diffuse axonal injury. Neural Regen Res 2015; 10(11):1879–81.

61. Rutman AM, Rapp EJ, Hippe DS, et al. T2*-weighted and diffusion magnetic resonance imaging differentiation of cerebral fat embolism from diffuse axonal injury. J Comput Assist Tomogr 2017;41(6):877–83.

62. Bodanapally UK, Shanmuganathan K, Saksobhavivat N, et al. MR imaging and differentiation of cerebral fat embolism syndrome from diffuse axonal injury: application of diffusion tensor imaging. Neuroradiology 2013;55(6):771–8.

63. Tong KA, Ashwal S, Holshouser BA, et al. Diffuse axonal injury in children: clinical correlation with hemorrhagic lesions. Ann Neurol 2004;56(1):36–50.

64. Huang YL, Kuo YS, Tseng YC, et al. Susceptibility-weighted MRI in mild traumatic brain injury. Neurology 2015;84(6):580–5.

65. Jarrett M, Tam R, Hernández-Torres E, et al. A prospective pilot investigation of brain volume, white matter hyperintensities, and hemorrhagic lesions after mild traumatic brain injury. Front Neurol 2016;7:11.

66. Lee JK, Wu J, Banks S, et al. Prevalence of traumatic findings on routine MRI in a large cohort of professional fighters. AJNR Am J Neuroradiol 2017;38(7): 1303–10.

67. Wang Y, Bartels HM, Nelson LD. A systematic review of ASL perfusion MRI in mild TBI. Neuropsychol Rev 2020. https://doi.org/10.1007/s11065-020-09451-7.

68. Lin CM, Tseng YC, Hsu HL, et al. Arterial spin labeling perfusion study in the patients with subacute mild traumatic brain injury. PLoS One 2016;11(2): e0149109.

69. Ge Y, Patel MB, Chen Q, et al. Assessment of thalamic perfusion in patients with mild traumatic brain injury by true FISP arterial spin labelling MR imaging at 3T. Brain Inj 2009;23(7–8):666–74.

70. Wang Y, Nelson LD, LaRoche AA, et al. Cerebral blood flow alterations in acute sport-related concussion. J Neurotrauma 2016;33(13):1227–36.

71. Len TK, Neary JP, Asmundson GJG, et al. Cerebrovascular reactivity impairment after sport-induced concussion. Med Sci Sports Exerc 2011;43(12): 2241–8.

72. Mutch WAC, Ellis MJ, Ryner LN, et al. Brain magnetic resonance imaging CO2 stress testing in adolescent postconcussion syndrome. J Neurosurg 2016;125(3):648–60.

73. Ross DE. Review of longitudinal studies of MRI brain volumetry in patients with traumatic brain injury. Brain Inj 2011;25(13–14):1271–8.

74. Bernick C, Banks SJ, Shin W, et al. Repeated head trauma is associated with smaller thalamic volumes and slower processing speed: the Professional Fighters' Brain Health Study. Br J Sports Med 2015;49(15):1007–11.

75. Singh R, Meier TB, Kuplicki R, et al. Relationship of collegiate football experience and concussion with hippocampal volume and cognitive outcomes. JAMA 2014;311(18):1883–8.

76. Koerte IK, Mayinger M, Muehlmann M, et al. Cortical thinning in former professional soccer players. Brain Imaging Behav 2016;10(3):792–8.

77. Bigler ED. Volumetric MRI findings in mild traumatic brain injury (mTBI) and neuropsychological outcome. Neuropsychol Rev 2021. https://doi.org/10.1007/s11065-020-09474-0.

78. Cole JH, Jolly A, de Simoni S, et al. Spatial patterns of progressive brain volume loss after moderate-severe traumatic brain injury. Brain 2018;141(3):822–36.

Clinical Updates in Mild Traumatic Brain Injury (Concussion)

Megan Moore, CRNP[a], Danielle K. Sandsmark, MD, PhD[b],*

KEYWORDS

• Concussion • Traumatic brain injury • Post-concussion syndrome

KEY POINTS

- Traumatic brain injury (TBI) is a common problem that leaves many with long-standing and life-altering deficits.
- Persistent post-TBI symptoms most commonly include headaches, sleep disruptions, vestibular and vision disturbances, mood changes, and cognitive dysfunction.
- Recognition of mild TBI (concussion) is important to initiate treatment strategies early after injury.

EPIDEMIOLOGY

Traumatic brain injury (TBI) is broadly defined as any disruption of brain function and/or structure due to an external physical force. More specifically, the Centers for Disease Control and Prevention (CDC), which perform surveillance monitoring of trauma-related injuries in the United States, define TBI as any blunt or penetrating trauma or from acceleration/deceleration forces that result in one or more of the following symptoms or signs: decreased level of consciousness, amnesia, skull fracture, intracranial lesion (most typically hemorrhage in one or more intracranial compartments), or objective neurologic or neuropsychological abnormality. Practically, non-penetrating and penetrating TBIs (such as those caused by ballistics) are thought to represent distinct pathologies. In this article, we focus on non-penetrating TBIs, which represent most of the trauma-related brain insults and have been the most rigorously studied.

The most recent comprehensive surveillance data from the CDC published in 2019 estimates 2.87 million emergency department visits, hospitalizations, and deaths in the United States annually related to TBI.[1] This represents a 53% increase from the prior report published in 2010.[2] These numbers do not include those who did not seek care or were cared for outside of a hospital setting, such as a primary care physician's office. Although the exact number of these injuries not evaluated in the hospital is unclear, they are estimated to represent 20% to 50% of mild TBIs.[3,4] Rates of TBI per 100,000 individuals remain highest among the elderly (>75 years old), the very young (0 to 4 years), and teens/young adults (aged 15 to 24 years). Although this age distribution is consistent with prior trends, there was a significant increase in fall-related injuries in the 2019 report, with fall-related TBIs increasing more than 80% from the prior report. This trend is thought to reflect our aging population and an increase in anticoagulation use and suggests that public health education and interventions related to fall prevention may be particularly important in the coming years.

Although there is an overall increase in the number of individuals with TBI being evaluated in hospital settings, the rate of hospital admissions for TBI actually decreased by 8% during the same

[a] Department of Neurology, University of Pennsylvania Perelman School of Medicine, 51 North 39th Street, Andrew Mutch Building 4th Floor, Philadelphia, PA 19104, USA; [b] Department of Neurology, Division of Neurocritical Care, University of Pennsylvania Perelman School of Medicine, 51 North 39th Street, Medical Office Building Suite 205, Philadelphia, PA 19104, USA
* Corresponding author.
E-mail address: Danielle.sandsmark@pennmedicine.upenn.edu

Neuroimag Clin N Am 33 (2023) 271–278
https://doi.org/10.1016/j.nic.2023.01.003

neuroimaging.theclinics.com

time period after age adjustment.[5] This decrease has been most dramatic as it relates to motor vehicle crashes (MVC), for which there was a 34% decrease in MVC-related TBI hospitalizations. Similarly, although the total number of MVC-related TBI deaths rose, the age-adjusted rates decreased by 6%. This is largely the reflection of public safety campaigns (eg, seat-belt and cell phone usage laws) and an improvement in vehicle safety features that have decreased the severity of primary TBI-related injury, rather than in changes in clinical management.

In the general population, TBI affects males more often than females. However, in sports-related injuries, females outnumber males. This is thought to be due to discrepancies in reporting as well as physiologic differences including head:-neck ratio. TBI comprises 10% to 15% of all sports-related injuries. American football leads the incidence of TBI, followed by women's soccer. This data is impacted by reporting inconsistencies across sports with varying degrees of impact.[6]

Beyond the acute injury, TBI is also a major public health concern not only because of the number of people affected, but also due to the long-term medical and socioeconomic costs, particularly for those who sustain injuries when they are young. Although prevalence estimate data are scarce, the CDC estimated that 2% of the population lived with chronic disability related to a TBI.[7] Given that these injuries occur frequently in younger people, this has a significant socioeconomic impact due to lost work productivity not only for TBI survivors but also for their caregivers. Care-related costs are also significant, particularly given that so many are injured at a young age. In fact, 74% of all years life lost due to TBI occur in affected individual's age groups with the potential to work (15 to 64 years).[8] In 2010, the annual costs of TBI in Europe were estimated to be 36.8 billion dollars (approximately $9820/individual).[9] Direct health care accounted for only 31% of these costs, 59% represented indirect costs related to productivity losses and other societal costs, and 10% represented indirect medical costs, such as nursing facilities. Globally, TBI is estimated to cost $400 billion annually.[10] This loss in productivity is not limited to those with the most severe insults. Recent data indicate that even in those with mild injuries, 17% of individuals were not working 1 year after injury and 21% reported a decrease in income.[1] Of those who had mild injuries and normal head imaging at the time of being seen in the emergency department, 35% had functional limitations 12 months post-injury.[5]

Many of the epidemiologic studies of recovery after "mild TBI" have focused on sports-related concussions. However, how applicable these injuries in physically active, typically younger adults to injuries sustained by a broader, generally older adult population sustaining injuries in motor vehicle accidents, falls, assault, or any other of a myriad of possible injuries, is unknown. Recently, Madhok and colleagues examined 991 subjects who presented to the ER with concussion (Glasgow Coma Score [GCS] = 15, negative head CT imaging) and enrolled in the TRACK-TBI observational study. Examining clinical outcomes 6 months after injury, they found that only 44% of individuals had recovered fully. These individuals reported deficits in work and social functioning, disruptions in family and friend relationships, and inability to return to pre-injury life. These problems were worse in those with known psychiatric co-morbidities, such as anxiety and depression, a finding that has been noted consistently in TBI studies.

Awareness of these ongoing deficits affecting the majority of individuals who present to the ER with this complaint is critical for their treating providers. Studies have shown that prompt referral following an ER presentation for concussion for mental health support and other therapies can improve outcomes.[11,12] Proper education can also help individuals set realistic and achievable goals in their recovery, as unrealistic expectations can lead to further distress and anxiety that exacerbate the experience of symptoms.[12]

Traumatic Brain Injury Classification

TBI is generally classified as mild, moderate, or severe, based on presenting GCS values. The GCS is scored based on the post-resuscitation in verbal, eye movement, and motor abilities and has a minimum score of 3, for someone in coma with no responses in any of the 3 domains, to a full score of 15, which reflects full consciousness and ability to participate in the neurologic examination. Of note, neuroimaging findings are not included in this classification scheme.

A TBI is classified as "mild" when an individual presents to clinical care with a GCS of 13 to 15. Mild TBI, which is often used synonymously with concussion, accounts for approximately 75% to 80% of all TBIs reported as well as the vast majority that go unreported. The term "mild" is a source of frustration for clinicians, patients, and families, as this grading system, intended purely for acute classification, does not take into consideration the diversity and severity of post-traumatic symptoms and the burden they may cause. Clinicians must often reassure patients that although their injury is technically considered mild, this classification may not accurately reflect the impact of their symptoms on daily functioning.

Since the initial adopting of the GCS score, various other clinical factors have been shown to factor into the likelihood of persistent symptoms following TBI, though none of these are formally included in the classification system. An injury characterized by loss of consciousness (LOC) and/or post-traumatic amnesia (PTA) is more likely to be associated with longer and more complicated recovery. Katz and Alexander[13] found a correlation between the duration of LOC and PTA and neurologic outcome, with longer durations of both LOC and PTA associated with worse Glasgow Outcome Scale scores at 6 and 12 months.

To provide synergy with other published literature, we will use the term mild TBI throughout this article to refer to injuries where consciousness is generally retained or quick to recover and there are no focal or objective neurologic deficits. It should be noted that mild TBI can be associated with trauma-induced neuroimaging changes, such as small contusions, subdural hemorrhages, or subarachnoid bleeding; these injuries are sometimes referred to as "complicated mild TBI", though none of the usual clinical classification tools use head computed tomography (CT) findings as part of TBI severity classification.

In the emergency department setting, mild TBIs are often missed as other more significant (and visible) injuries take priority. Frequently, patients are discharged home without any official diagnosis of TBI nor symptoms or management education.[14] Symptoms of neurologic dysfunction may not fully manifest until individuals resume work or life activities. Only then may it become obvious that they are experiencing cognitive, vestibular, mood, or headache-related symptoms. Lack of clearly defined diagnostic criteria for mild TBI leads to underreporting, delayed intervention, and missed care completely. In the outpatient setting, patients often present months after their injury having not realized they suffered a TBI. This can lead to prolonged post-traumatic symptoms that are more refractory to treatment as the patients have struggled to manage on their own without proper intervention.

Clinical Symptoms/Problems

Epidemiologic studies suggest that 80% of individuals who sustain a mild TBI will recover within 14 days.[5] These data are largely drawn from sports-related concussions and thus tend to be from studies of relatively young and active individuals. Although there are fewer studies in older and more diverse clinical populations, what data are available indicate that complete recovery following a mild TBI is similar to that observed in sports-related concussion.[5]

Given the sheer number of individuals who sustain a mild TBI each year, even 20% of individuals with longer-term symptoms represent a significant medical need. Unfortunately, the trajectory of care for these individuals is rarely clear. They are often referred to their primary care provider. Occasionally they will be seen by neurosurgery, neurology, or physical medicine and rehabilitation. However, the referral to outpatient care tends to be highly variable, both in terms of the type of specialist referred to and even if the referral happens at all. This can lead to delays in care that may ultimately compromise or extend the recovery period. Furthermore, therapies provided by specially trained physical, occupational, and speech/cognitive therapists is often indicated, but may be difficult for individuals to seek out and not all providers may be aware of these resources. All of these variables can result in delays of care.

Symptoms following TBI vary widely across the patient population. There are several common post-traumatic symptoms for which patients seek care in the weeks to months after their injury: headaches, cognitive problems, mood disturbance, sleep disturbance, and vestibular/vision dysfunction (Fig. 1). The various symptoms affect our heterogeneous patient population in different ways. Patients who are very high functioning before their injury will be more disrupted by seemingly minor cognitive symptoms than those for whom critical thinking and communicating are not as essential. Those who had preexisting pain, mood, or vestibular dysfunction may see those problems amplified following injury.

The ability to modify activity—physical, emotional, and mental—during the weeks following a TBI greatly impacts one's recovery. Previously, the backbone of post-TBI care was to prescribe "brain rest" for an ill-defined period of time, typically until symptoms were completely or largely resolved. Given the subjective nature of post-TBI symptoms, implementation and adherence was highly variable. Finally, this was studied in a randomized controlled trial of teenagers who sustained sports-related concussions.[15] Groups were randomized to either 10 days of complete cognitive and physical rest, or graduated return to normal activities. Actigraphy allowed researchers to monitor individuals' movement and sleep. Although the investigators had hypothesized that cognitive rest would improve outcomes, they actually found the opposite: those in the brain rest group had more post-concussive symptoms and worse cognitive performance at 10 days post-injury. Those in the strict rest group also

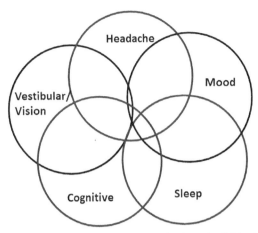

Fig. 1. Symptoms experienced by individuals following a mild TBI/concussion frequently occur in these domains. Symptoms that persist are typically most prominent in one to two domains though all may be present to varying degrees early following injury. Symptoms are frequently interconnected and must therefore be addressed in a stepwise fashion.

reported more emotional symptoms. Based on these data, we recommend a period of 24 to 48 h of relative rest and then a gradual return to some activities, as symptoms allow.

When counseling patients on resuming work/school, a graduated schedule provides the foundation for a more successful return to pre-injury activity level. Being able to limit total daily hours and days per week and slowly increase as tolerated helps patients navigate normalizing their activity. Patients often struggle if they are expected to produce 8- or 12-h worth of work in 4 or 6 h, so emphasizing that a time limitation includes limiting productivity expectations is important. Limiting workplace and other distractions have been identified as an important target area.[16] Other accommodations to consider include limiting the total number of tasks or projects, allowing for scheduled breaks throughout the day, extensions for due dates, and environment modifications to decrease stimulation.

As providers, we need to work with our patients and develop management strategies that are relevant, able to be implemented, accessible, and do not add to stress or burden. In our experience, it is important to recommend a stepwise framework for treatment and therapy, as executing numerous different recommendations can be overwhelming. It is often most beneficial to prioritize symptom management in one domain at the first visit with a plan for short-interval follow-up to further explore other issues. Patients frequently find that improving one area of concern will indirectly lessen the burden of other areas.

Current Treatment Strategies

Clinical management of TBI is both an art and a science. Recent increase in awareness has propelled research funding to better understand the clinical features and epidemiology of mild TBI, but research related to treatment interventions is lacking in the area of mild TBI. Because 80% of individuals get better without any intervention, such trials require large sample sizes or careful selection of subsets of patients. Because it is currently not possible to identify those at the highest risk of poorer outcomes, participant selection for such trials has not been feasible. Large observational studies are now underway and are giving us an initial sense of long-term outcomes in these populations. Some of these trials are just beginning and a large component of patient education should center on the prevention of further brain injuries and promotion of cerebrovascular health.

Post-traumatic headaches

Post-traumatic headaches share many features of migraine and tension headaches. Therefore, treatment is approached similarly to those primary headache disorders, using a tiered approach. Depending on the frequency and severity of headaches, abortive versus prophylactic strategies can be explored. Abortive therapies include over-the-counter analgesics such as acetaminophen, ibuprofen, and naproxen. NSAIDs should be avoided for a short period if any intracranial bleeding is identified; however, the exact time period to abstain from these medications is unclear. A combination of acetaminophen, aspirin, and caffeine such as Excedrin Migraine is often better than any sole agent. Escalation to prescription abortive agents, such as triptans, antiemetics, and calcitonin gene-related peptide (CGRP) antagonists can be implemented when over-the-counter (OTC) treatments are ineffective. To prevent medication overuse headache, OTC analgesics, like acetaminophen and ibuprofen, should be limited to no more than 3 days' use per week. If OTCs are ineffective, prescription prophylactic medications that are taken daily and intended for headache prevention should be started. The first lines of treatment can include selective serotonin reuptake inhibitors (SSRIs), serotonin and norepinephrine reuptake inhibitors (SNRIs), anti-epileptic agents, calcium channel blockers, and beta-blockers. We typically try to use agents that correlate with other symptoms the patient is experiencing (eg, tricyclic antidepressants if the patient is also experiencing neuropathic pain or sleep disturbance). Consideration for referral to headache specialist for intractable migraine treatment can be considered if needed.

There are several vitamin supplements that have data supporting their use for headache prevention including magnesium, riboflavin, and CoQ10. Most of these data derive from studies of migraine headaches,[17] but can be trialed for the prevention of ongoing post-traumatic headaches.

There is frequently a contribution from cervical neck pain that contributes to headaches in patients following mild TBI, particularly those who sustain whiplash-like injuries. Early referral to physical therapy for treatment of neck pain which may be contributing to the sensation of headache should be considered early, and can often be coupled with vestibular physical therapy, discussed below.

Sleep disturbance

Good quality sleep is essential for brain injury recovery and overall health maintenance. During sleep, the brain sleep disturbance occurs due to disruption of the cellular environment, hormonal fluctuations, and interference with homeostasis. Physical and psychological post-traumatic symptoms can also affect sleep. Sleep deprivation has been shown to affect long-term recovery in TBI patients, and can contribute to accelerated neurodegeneration.[18] Poor quality sleep is associated with higher levels of anxiety, depression, posttraumatic stress, pain, memory performance, and attention. Implementation of high-quality sleep hygiene, mindfulness, and optimizing management of physical and psychological symptoms will promote better sleep. Melatonin supplementation can be helpful in re-establishing the sleep-wake cycle. Using pharmacologic sleep aids can be helpful in certain situations where appropriate within the total clinical picture. Referral to psychology for cognitive behavioral therapy for insomnia (CBT-I) is often beneficial.[19]

Vestibular dysfunction

Vestibular dysfunction can be particularly disabling for patients and is predictive of those who go on to have prolonged symptoms.[20] Vestibular dysfunction can manifest in a variety of ways. Gait disturbance may be prominent early on, but persistent deficits tend to be more subtle. Patients may describe a sensation of feeling unsteady, but rarely report true vertigo. Movement may worsen symptoms. Vestibular disturbances frequently overlap with visual tracking dysfunction.[21] Gaze stabilization is frequently affected and often manifests as difficulty with reading, driving, watching television, or navigating computer/phone screens. Patients may report worsening headaches or other pain after periods of these activities. This can be particularly problematic for individuals upon returning to work when using computer screens for extended periods. These problems can be present even in the absence of frank gait disturbance or eye-tracking abnormalities on bedside testing.

Referral to physical and occupational therapists who specialize in neurorehabilitation and vestibular therapy should be pursued relatively early if symptoms persist beyond 1 month. Vision therapy, generally performed by optometrists, can also be pursued. Although the data is limited, vision therapy for convergence and accommodative inefficiencies can be effective in a subset of patients.[22] In our experience, this therapy is less likely to be covered by insurance. Therefore, we frequently refer to vestibular physical therapy first and refer to vision therapy only if that is not effective in relieving symptoms. We have had frequent success with this approach.

Mood disturbance

The frontal lobes of the brain are uniquely susceptible to TBI, which may be one reason why mood disturbances, particularly depression and anxiety, are common following TBI. In addition, the traumatic events surrounding the injury can predispose individuals to anxiety and other posttraumatic stress. Individuals with preexisting depression and anxiety, whether diagnosed or not, are known to have a poorer recovery following TBI.[23] A careful history to determine prior symptoms of or diagnosed mood disorder is essential. Referral to psychology to establish counseling/talk therapy is appropriate in addition to connecting patients to mindfulness resources. In some cases, mood stabilizers, antidepressants, or anxiolytics should be considered.

Cognitive dysfunction

Cognitive dysfunction in the TBI population often presents with short-term memory impairment, difficulty concentrating and focusing, executive dysfunction, and word-finding difficulty. Cognitive dysfunction is typically multi-factorial and impacted by the symptoms described above: poorly controlled headaches, sleep disruptions, and mood disturbances all contribute to a sensation of poor cognitive performance. Efforts to address these issues should commence before (or at least in sync with) referral to cognitive therapy, often performed by a specially trained speech pathologist. Comprehensive TBI rehabilitation programs can accommodate this skilled therapy.

If it has been at least 6 months from injury and after participating in cognitive therapy a patient continues to experience disruptive cognitive symptoms, referral to neuropsychology is appropriate. Neuropsychological evaluation can flush out the nuances of cognitive dysfunction and determine more specific contributing factors, which may include mood disturbances, anxiety, neurodegenerative disorders, or attention-deficit disorders. Targeting treatment strategies to specific causes of symptoms increases the potential for recovery. Neuropsychological testing performed while a patient is acutely symptomatic in the early stages of recovery may not yield reliable results, so it is important to optimize the management of other symptoms (headache, dizziness, mood) before referral.

Long-Term Outcomes Following Traumatic Brain Injury

As mentioned, most individuals with mild TBI will recover fully. Although our clinical experience is that the above approach to treatment helps the 20% with persistent symptoms, these interventions have not been systematically studied in a TBI population with robust attention to recovery outcomes. Furthermore, the temporal relationship of these interventions to clinical recovery is not understood. Our clinical experience indicates a wide variability in the recovery timeline, but the overall trajectory is generally one of improvement. Moreover, these therapies can be effective even long after the initial injury. Occasionally, therapies will need to be revisited when symptoms worsen, almost always in the setting of a stressor or repeat injury.

One of the most feared long-term consequences of TBI is progressive cognitive decline and dementia, which typically presents years to decades after brain injury. It has long been recognized that moderate and severe TBI in early and mid-life is associated with an increased risk of late-life dementia, with relative risks on the order of 2.5 to 5.0.[24–29] More recently, it has become evident that even milder injuries are associated with an increased risk of later-life cognitive decline and dementia. These studies, performed in diverse populations across the lifespan, show significant associations, with hazard ratios of 1.5 to 3.8, of TBI of any severity with the development of later dementia.[25,27,28,30–33] Moreover, individuals with TBI present for dementia evaluations more than their non-injured peers.[34] Even the mildest form of traumatic brain insults, TBI without LOC, was associated with an increased risk of dementia (hazard ratio [HR] 2.36; confidence interval [CI] 2.06 to 2.36) compared with an age-matched, non-TBI veteran control group.[24] Recently, these findings were confirmed in a large, observational cohort study in which over 14,000 adults were followed over 25 years.[33] In the study,

investigators found that any mild head injury was associated with a hazard ratio of 1.44 for the development of dementia compared with non-injured participants. These associations increased with the number of head injuries and were stronger in female and white participants. Although the injuries captured in this study likely do not reflect the mildest injuries (as self-reported injuries required LOC), they raise a concern about the risk of these injuries contributing to cognitive decline later in life.

Future Needs in Clinical Care of Mild Traumatic Brain Injury/Concussion

Important steps have been made in the last decade to recognize mild TBIs and the impacts that mild TBI can have on long-term functioning. In 2018, the first biomarkers for the distinction of mild TBI associated with intracranial hemorrhage were approved by the FDA.[35] However, the penetration of these biomarkers into clinical use has been limited. Studies to develop point-of-care assays that can be used for clinical decision-making at the bedside are ongoing. One major limitation of these biomarkers is that they are not yet shown to correlate with long-term outcomes. Ultimately, to design appropriately powered clinical trials, we will need biomarkers—which may include blood, physiologic testing, or neuroimaging—that can help us to distinguish the 80% of individuals with mild TBI who will get better on their own from the 20% who develop longer term and disabling symptoms or from those who develop later cognitive decline and dementia. By being able to distinguish these groups, we will be able to enroll individuals that are most likely to benefit from new therapies. Ongoing observational studies[5,36] that include detailed acute injury phenotyping, biomarker collection, and long-term follow-up will be key to developing acute biomarkers that are predictive of later recovery.

CLINICS CARE POINTS

- A brief period (24–48 hours) of rest following a mild TBI is reasonable; longer periods of complete inactivity are likely counterproductive.
- Assess patients at each post-concussive visit for headaches, sleep disturbances, vestibular and visual dysfunction, mood disturbances, and cognitive dysfunction.
- Symptoms lasting >2–4 weeks warrant referral for additional therapy and/or medication trial.

DISCLOSURE

The authors report no financial or commercial conflicts of interest. Dr D.K. Sandsmark receives funding from the National Institute of Neurological Disorders and Stroke (K23- NS104239).

REFERENCES

1. Centers for Disease Control and Prevention. Surveillance report of traumatic brain injury-related emergency department visits, hospitalizations, and deaths—United States, 2014. Atlanta, GA: Centers for Disease Control and Prevention, U.S. Department of Health and Human Services; 2019.
2. CDC C for DC and P. Rates of TBI-related emergency department visits, hospitalizations, and deaths: United States, 2001 – 2010 | data. Atlanta, GA: Centers for Disease Control and Prevention; 2010.
3. Thorne J, Markovic S, Chih H, et al. Healthcare choices following mild traumatic brain injury in Australia. BMC Health Serv Res 2022;22(1):858.
4. Setnik L, Bazarian JJ. The characteristics of patients who do not seek medical treatment for traumatic brain injury. Brain Inj 2007;21(1):1–9.
5. Madhok DY, Rodriguez RM, Barber J, et al. Outcomes in Patients With Mild Traumatic Brain Injury Without Acute Intracranial Traumatic Injury. JAMA Netw Open 2022;5(8):e2223245.
6. Capizzi A, Woo J, Verduzco-Gutierrez M. Traumatic Brain Injury: An Overview of Epidemiology, Pathophysiology, and Medical Management. Med Clin North Am 2020;104(2):213–38.
7. Center for Disease Control and Prevention. Traumatic Brain Injury in the United States: A Report to Congress. 1999. Available at: https://www.cdc.gov/traumaticbraininjury/pdf/TBI_in_the_US.pdf.
8. Majdan M, Plancikova D, Maas A, et al. Years of life lost due to traumatic brain injury in Europe: A cross-sectional analysis of 16 countries. Plos Med 2017, 14(7):e1002331.
9. Norup A, Kruse M, Soendergaard PL, et al. Socioeconomic Consequences of Traumatic Brain Injury: A Danish Nationwide Register-Based Study. J Neurotrauma 2020;37(24):2694–702.
10. Maas AIR, Menon DK, Adelson PD, et al. Traumatic brain injury: integrated approaches to improve prevention, clinical care, and research. Lancet Neurol 2017. https://doi.org/10.1016/S1474-4422(17)30371-X. Published online.
11. Tiersky LA, Anselmi V, Johnston MV, et al. A Trial of Neuropsychologic Rehabilitation in Mild-Spectrum Traumatic Brain Injury. Arch Phys Med Rehabil 2005;86(8):1565–74.
12. Ponsford J, Willmott C, Rothwell A, et al. Impact of early intervention on outcome following mild head injury in adults. J Neurol Neurosurg Psychiatr 2002;73(3):330–2.
13. Katz DI, Alexander MP. Traumatic Brain Injury: Predicting Course of Recovery and Outcome for Patients Admitted to Rehabilitation. Arch Neurol 1994; 51(7):661–70.
14. Seabury SA, Gaudette É, Goldman DP, et al. Assessment of Follow-up Care After Emergency Department Presentation for Mild Traumatic Brain Injury and Concussion: Results From the TRACK-TBI Study. JAMA Netw Open 2018;1(1):e180210.
15. Thomas DG, Apps JN, Hoffmann RG, et al. Benefits of strict rest after acute concussion: a randomized controlled trial. Pediatrics 2015;135(2):213–23.
16. Pinnow D, Causey-Upton R, Meulenbroek P. Navigating the impact of workplace distractions for persons with TBI: a qualitative descriptive study. Sci Rep 2022;12:15881.
17. Schwedt TJ. Preventive Therapy of Migraine. Continuum (Minneap Minn) 2018;24(4, Headache): 1052–65.
18. Barshikar S, Bell KR. Sleep Disturbance After TBI. Curr Neurol Neurosci Rep 2017;17(11):87.
19. Ymer L, McKay A, Wong D, et al. Cognitive Behavioral Therapy for Sleep Disturbance and Fatigue Following Acquired Brain Injury: Predictors of Treatment Response. J Head Trauma Rehabil 2022;37(3): E220–30.
20. Master CL, Master SR, Wiebe DJ, et al. Vision and Vestibular System Dysfunction Predicts Prolonged Concussion Recovery in Children. Clin J Sport Med 2018;28(2):139–45.
21. Xiang L, Bansal S, Wu AY, et al. Pathway of care for visual and vestibular rehabilitation after mild traumatic brain injury: a critical review. Brain Inj 2022; 36(8):911–20.
22. Gallaway M, Scheiman M, Mitchell GL. Vision Therapy for Post-Concussion Vision Disorders. Optom Vis Sci 2017;94(1):68–73.
23. McCauley SR, Boake C, Levin HS, et al. Postconcussional Disorder Following Mild to Moderate Traumatic Brain Injury: Anxiety, Depression, and Social Support as Risk Factors and Comorbidities. J Clin Exp Neuropsychol 2001;23(6):792–808.
24. Barnes DE, Byers AL, Gardner RC, et al. Association of mild traumatic brain injury with and without loss of consciousness with dementia in US military veterans. JAMA Neurol 2018;75(9):1055.
25. Gardner RC, Burke JF, Nettiksimmons J, et al. Dementia risk after traumatic brain injury vs nonbrain trauma: The role of age and severity. JAMA Neurol 2014;71(12):1490–7.
26. Barnes DE, Kaup A, Kirby KA, et al. Traumatic brain injury and risk of dementia in older veterans. J Emerg Med 2014;47(5):617–8.
27. Nordström P, Michaëlsson K, Gustafson Y, et al. Traumatic brain injury and young onset dementia:

A nationwide cohort study. Ann Neurol 2014;75(3): 374–81.

28. Fann JR, Ribe AR, Pedersen HS, et al. Long-term risk of dementia among people with traumatic brain injury in Denmark: a population-based observational cohort study. Lancet Psychiatry 2018;5(5):424–31.

29. Hof PR, Bouras C, Buée L, et al. Differential distribution of neurofibrillary tangles in the cerebral cortex of dementia pugilistica and Alzheimer's disease cases. Acta neuropathologica 1992;85(1):23–30.

30. Lee YK, Hou SW, Lee CC, et al. Increased risk of dementia in patients with mild traumatic brain injury: a nationwide cohort study. PloS one 2013;8(5): e62422. Zhang XY, ed.

31. Dams-O'Connor K, Gibbons LE, Bowen JD, et al. Risk for late-life re-injury, dementia and death among individuals with traumatic brain injury: a population-based study. J Neurol Neurosurg Psychiatr 2013;84(2):177–82.

32. Gardner RC, Langa KM, Yaffe K. Subjective and objective cognitive function among older adults with a history of traumatic brain injury: A population-based cohort study. PLoS Med 2017; 14(3):1–16.

33. Schneider ALC, Selvin E, Latour L, et al. Head injury and 25-year risk of dementia. Alzheimers Dement 2021;17(9):1432–41.

34. Iacono D, Raiciulescu S, Olsen C, et al. Traumatic brain injury exposure lowers age of cognitive decline in AD and non-AD conditions. Front Neurol 2021;12.

35. Bazarian JJ, Biberthaler P, Welch RD, et al. Serum GFAP and UCH-L1 for prediction of absence of intracranial injuries on head CT (ALERT-TBI): a multicentre observational study. Lancet Neurol 2018; 17(9):782–9.

36. Voormolen DC, Zeldovich M, Haagsma JA, et al. Outcomes after Complicated and Uncomplicated Mild Traumatic Brain Injury at Three-and Six-Months Post-Injury: Results from the CENTER-TBI Study. J Clin Med 2020;9(5):1525.

Current State of Diffusion-Weighted Imaging and Diffusion Tensor Imaging for Traumatic Brain Injury Prognostication

Matthew Grant, MD[a,b,c,]*, JiaJing Liu, MD, PhD[a], Max Wintermark, MD[a,d],
Ulas Bagci, PhD[e,f], David Douglas, MD[a,g]

KEYWORDS

- Traumatic brain injury (TBI) • Concussion • Diffusion tensor imaging (DTI) • Kurtosis • Anisotropy
- MR imaging • Prognosis • Machine learning (ML)

KEY POINTS

- Diffusion tensor imaging (DTI) generally shows low fractional anisotropy (FA) and high mean diffusivity (MD) values in patients with TBI-related injury. However, many diseases can also show altered FA and MD values. Results should therefore be interpreted with caution and in the full clinical context.
- A key limitation of DTI is its inability to resolve crossing white matter tract fibers within a voxel. Advanced techniques, such as diffusion kurtosis imaging (DKI), can better resolve this at the expense of increased imaging time and more involved computing.
- Although research shows a general trend toward low FA values in TBI patients, this can only be said at the group level and exact cutoffs differentiating normal versus abnormal have not yet been established to allow these data to be applied to individual patients. Future research will better clarify this.

INTRODUCTION

Traumatic brain injury (TBI) occurs when a penetrating or blunt traumatic injury disrupts the normal function of the brain.[1] In the United States, TBI annually affects over 1.7 million people, resulting in approximately 224,000 hospitalizations and 61,000 deaths, although the exact incidence is unknown.[2-5] Furthermore, nearly 3 million US residents are living with mild to severe long-term disability from TBI, with symptoms such as headache, depression, cognitive impairment, post-traumatic stress disorder, and visual disturbances.[6,7] The estimated annual cost of non-fatal TBI in the United States is $40.5 billion.[8]

TBI can occur from a wide range of mechanisms with the most common causes including motor vehicle accidents, falls, sports-related injuries, suicide, and assault.[2-4] Among civilians, falls are the most common cause of TBI overall (nearly 50%

[a] Department of Radiology, Stanford University, 453 Quarry Road, Palo Alto, CA 94304, USA; [b] Department of Radiology, Uniformed Services University of the Health Sciences, 4301 Jones Bridge Rd, Bethesda, MD 20814, USA; [c] Department of Radiology, Landstuhl Regional Medical Center, Dr Hitzelberger Straße, 66849 Landstuhl, Germany; [d] Neuroradiology Department, The University of Texas Anderson Cancer Center, 1400 Pressler Street, Unit 1482, Houston, TX 77030, USA; [e] Radiology and Biomedical Engineering Department, Northwestern University, 737 North Michigan Drive, Suite 1600, Chicago, IL 60611, USA; [f] Department of Computer Science, University of Central Florida, 4328 Scorpius Street, Orlando, Florida, 32816; [g] Department of Radiology, 96th Medical Group, Eglin Air Force Base, 307 Boatner Road, Eglin Air Force Base, Florida 32542, USA
* Corresponding author. 453 Quarry Road, Palo Alto, CA 94304.
E-mail address: mgrant84@stanford.edu

Neuroimag Clin N Am 33 (2023) 279–297
https://doi.org/10.1016/j.nic.2023.01.004

in 2017) whereas suicide is the most common cause of TBI-related deaths (34.7% in 2017).[2,5] Men are much more affected than women and the elderly are much more affected by falls.[5] Specific to the military population, common causes also include penetrating and blast-related injury.[9]

TBI chronicity can be classified as acute (less than 2 weeks), subacute (2 weeks to 1 year), or chronic (greater than 1 year).[10] The severity of TBI in the acute setting can be assessed using the Glasgow Coma Scale (GCS), which is a 15-point scale that combines eye opening (1–4 points), motor response (1–6 points), and verbal response (1–5 points). GCS scores of 13 to 15, 9 to 12, and, 3 to 8, define mild, moderate, and severe TBI, respectively.[11] However, the long-term prognostic ability of the GCS is limited and a better quantitative approach is urgently needed.[12] In this regard, neuroimaging plays a critical role in the diagnosis and management of TBI. In the acute setting, for example, the role of conventional computed tomography (CT) and MR imaging in identifying injuries that require acute neurosurgical management is well established. However, in the setting of mild traumatic brain injury (mTBI), also referred to as "concussion," these modalities often depict normal anatomy and therefore lack sensitivity in diagnosis and prognosis.[13] Even when an abnormality is visible by conventional imaging, the full extent of the injury may not be completely demonstrated. Therefore, it remains challenging to predict outcomes from first-line clinical tools and conventional neuroimaging approaches. Advanced imaging techniques are needed not only to accurately diagnose injury severity, but also to provide prognostic information, assist with clinical management, and guide clinical trials of novel therapeutic agents.

Compared with conventional MR imaging and CT, diffusion tensor imaging (DTI) is an advanced MR imaging technique that has been applied to study a range of clinical conditions, including TBI, and complements the available neuroimaging approaches in multiple promising aspects.[14–16] The purpose of this article is to review the current state of DTI and its relationship to prognosis in TBI. Conventional imaging and clinical management of TBI are discussed elsewhere in this issue. To this end, we will begin by briefly reviewing the principles underlying DTI, including its strengths and limitations. Next, we will provide an overview of the current scientific knowledge using DTI for prognostication in TBI, with an emphasis on brain white matter (WM) injury in mTBI. Last, we will conclude with a brief discussion on future directions regarding technological advances and areas of research.

TECHNIQUE

Before discussing the role of DTI in TBI prognosis, it is important to have a basic understanding of how diffusion images are acquired and assumptions that are made when imaging the brain. Many excellent books and review articles have been published discussing DTI in great detail.[17–22] Here, we will provide the reader with the most fundamental knowledge.

The human brain is composed of a variety of tissue types and can be grossly separated into gray matter (GM) and WM. WM is composed predominantly of axons, supporting tissues, and glial cells. Axons travel from GM, where the neuron cell bodies are located, to other areas of the brain or spinal cord via WM axons (also called *tracts*). Within the brain, axons connect neurons of different brain regions into functional circuits. Visualizing and quantifying WM and its tracts is a desirable tool to distinguish normal from the abnormal brain in mTBI. However, conventional MR imaging sequences (using both T1-weighted and T2-weighted sequences) are unable to visualize many of these WM tracts because contrast resolution in conventional MR imaging sequences is based solely on T1 and T2 relaxation times, which are similar in WM tracts regardless of direction.

Diffusion-weighted imaging (DWI), on the other hand, is routinely a spin-echo-based imaging sequence typically used in clinical practice and can help in identifying structural connectivity in the brain (Fig. 1). DWI uses one reference image (B = 0 s/mm^2) and one additional B-value (such as B = 1000 s/mm^2). In doing so, DWI can measure the movement of water within an imaged volume comprised of voxels. Water not diffusing out from its original voxel retains its signal and is characteristically bright on imaging, known as "restricted diffusion." To capture diffusivity regardless of direction, usually three orthogonally oriented diffusion gradients are used. DWI is useful in the diagnosis of a variety of conditions including brain tumors and stroke. However, a standard clinical DWI sequence does not provide information regarding the direction of diffusion.

DTI is a more advanced sequence than DWI because DTI uses more diffusion-sensitizing gradients and directions. At least two diffusion-sensitizing gradients in each x, y, and z directions are used with one reference image (B = 0 s/mm^2) and one additional B-value (such as B = 1000 s/mm^2) for a minimum of six gradients. When water diffuses equally in all directions, it is called "isotropic" diffusion. Likewise, if water preferentially diffuses in one direction, this is known as "anisotropic" diffusion. In WM tracts, barriers to

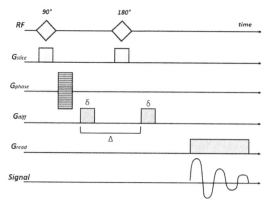

Fig. 1. Diagram showing the pulsed gradient spin-echo sequence used for DWI. Two diffusion-encoding gradients (G_{diff}) are added to the standard spin-echo sequence to create a phase shift proportional to the water displacement along the gradient direction. δ, duration of the diffusion-encoding gradient; Δ, diffusion time interval; G_{phase}, phase-encoding gradient; G_{read}, readout gradient; G_{slice}, slice-selection gradient; RF, radiofrequence pulse.

diffusion, such as cell membranes and myelin sheaths, contribute to anisotropy so that the diffusion direction of water occurs predominantly parallel with the axons, along the path of least resistance, and is restricted in the orthogonal direction (Fig. 2).[23]

In its simplest form, DTI can be illustrated with the Gaussian single tensor (single ellipsoid) model.[24,25] Although six is the minimum number of diffusion gradients used in DTI, by applying up to 30 or more diffusion-sensitizing gradients in multiple directions, DTI can better image the anisotropy of water diffusion and thereby improve visualization of WM tracts (Figs. 3 and 4).[19,21,22,26–29]

For each voxel, a set of directions and magnitudes forming a three-dimensional (3D) ellipsoid can be generated representing the tissue microenvironment. This 3D ellipsoid is characterized by three eigenvectors, which define the axes, and three associated eigenvalues (λ), which define the lengths. Axial diffusivity (AD) describes diffusion along the principal axis (principal eigenvector) of the diffusion ellipsoid, whereas radial diffusivity (RD) is an average of diffusion along its two minor axes. Two primary metrics in DTI are mean diffusivity (MD), the total amount of diffusion in a voxel, and fractional anisotropy (FA), the relative anisotropy in a voxel. MD is calculated as the average of the three eigenvalues whereas FA is calculated as the square root of the sum of squares of the diffusivity differences divided by the square root sum of squares of the diffusivities (Fig. 5).[30] FA

values range between 0 and 1 with a value of 0 describing a state of random Brownian water motion, and a value of 1 describing uniform diffusion along a single direction, neither of which is exactly encountered in tissue.[7] Graphically, FA can characterize the 3D ellipsoid as linear, planar, or spherical with an FA value of 0 (isotropic diffusion) appearing as a sphere and an FA of 1 would be represented by an infinite cylinder (Fig. 6).

The diffusion tensor model assumes that there is a single ellipsoid, modeling the water molecules' motion, with all axons traveling in the same direction within each imaging voxel. Although it is possible to produce an image that represents the diffusion ellipsoid in every voxel, routinely interpreting such an image would be difficult (see Fig. 14, column B, discussed later). Therefore, images are typically displayed in gray scale or color-coded maps, whereby color represents the principal eigenvector and intensity (brightness) represents the FA value (Fig. 7).[14,15,17–22,26,27] These maps provide a useful compromise between ease of interpretation and clinical utility. However, despite the appealing nature of the acquisition speed and simplicity of the technique, it is not without limitations which will be discussed later.

Diffusion tensor data can also be used to produce tractography maps, either at the regional or whole brain level.[10] For regional analysis, workstations allow one to select a region of interest (ROI) to select the fiber tracts of interest (Fig. 8). Criteria can be set to isolate the tract of interest such as excessive angular deviation of the fiber tracts (eg, 37°), subthreshold voxel anisotropy (eg, FA 0.2), minimum fiber length (eg, 50 mm), or if it passes through certain anatomic structures known to contain the tract of interest (eg, the internal capsule and cerebral peduncles in the corticospinal tracts).[31,32] Because the process of tract selection is highly interactive it can result in bias.

When performing DTI in clinical care or research, careful attention to acquisition and post-processing must be taken. Signal to noise ratio is optimal at 3 T MR imaging due to the signal strengths. A full discussion of acquisition parameters is outside the scope of this discussion, but standard protocol parameters have been previously described (Box 1).[29,33,34] Information more specific to research protocols has also been described elsewhere.[35]

WHITE MATTER CHANGES IN TRAUMATIC BRAIN INJURY

Although most applications of DTI in current clinical practice are used in pre-operative planning for tumor or epilepsy lesion resection, given its

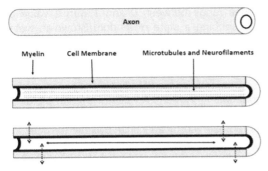

Fig. 2. Major barriers to diffusion in WM tracts include the cell membrane and myelin sheaths such that diffusion of water occurs predominantly parallel within the axon microtubules and neurofilaments, along the path of least resistance (*solid double arrow*), and is restricted in the orthogonal direction (*dashed arrows*).

ability to image WM tracts, there is great interest in performing DTI to assess axonal injury in TBI. In healthy WM, diffusion is constrained by the organization of axons, as previously discussed, and FA is generally high whereas MD is low. In the setting of TBI, however, WM, FA, and MD values can be altered, possibly indicating axonal injury. Many DTI researchers have studied TBI, primarily evaluating FA and MD, with widely variable results. The key factors affecting the imaging findings include the time between injury onset and imaging, the severity of the injury, and location of the injury within the brain (Fig. 9).

Concerning timing, in the acute period, an increase in FA and an overall decrease in diffusivity has been shown, possibly from cytotoxic edema after the injury.[36-38] However, many studies performed in the subacute or chronic time frames have found decreased FA and increased MD when compared with the control group.[37,39-57] The decreased FA is possibly due to demyelination or disruption of tissue microstructure.

Concerning severity, a recent meta-analysis of 44 studies was performed analyzing DTI changes in mild, moderate, and severe TBI in a large variety of brain regions.[58] In the mild TBI subgroup analysis, 88% of the brain regions examined had lower FA values when compared with the control group, whereas the moderate–severe TBI subgroup analysis showed 92% of the regions having lower FA values. For MD, 95% and 100% of the regions examined were higher in the TBI group than the control group for mild and moderate to severe TBI, respectively. Although this meta-analysis did not show any time-dependent changes, another study showed that after mTBI, the FA and diffusivity may normalize over time.[40,58] New evidence suggests that FA values may increase in both acute and chronic post-injury phases.[59] Variability in the data regarding the direction of TBI-related change may reflect heterogeneity within studied populations, including variation in TBI severity, injury location, imaging parameters, and imaging time from injury as discussed later.[59]

Concerning locations, specific locations of injury are also variable, which may be due to the heterogeneous nature of TBI. In subacute or chronic stages following mTBI, FA has been shown to be altered in several brain areas including midline structures such as the corpus callosum (CC), cingulum, and fornix, as well as the frontal lobes,

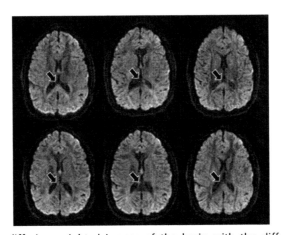

Fig. 3. Multiple transverse diffusion-weighted images of the brain with the diffusion gradients applied in different directions showing anisotropic diffusion. The signal intensity of WM varies with the direction of diffusion gradients, most notably in the CC (*arrows*). The signal is strongest when the diffusion gradient is oriented orthogonal to the WM fiber tracts (*upper right panel*) and weakest when the gradient is oriented parallel to the WM fiber tracts (*lower middle panel*).

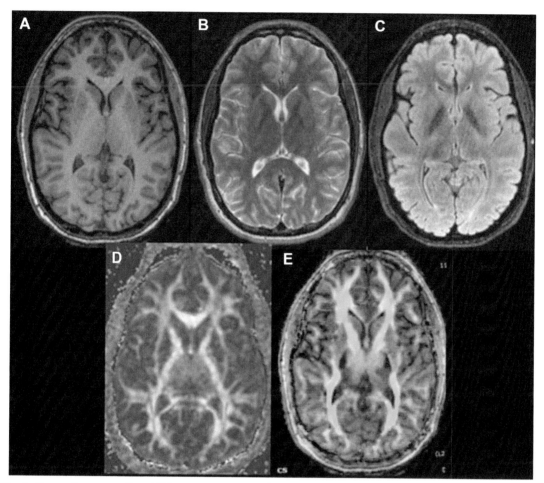

Fig. 4. Comparing conventional MR sequences to DTI. The top row shows that T1-weighted (*A*), T2-weighted (*B*), and T2-FLAIR (*C*) images of the brain cannot distinguish different fiber tracts given that WM tracts display similar signal intensity regardless of direction. The bottom row shows that DTI images can distinguish these tracts. Image (*D*) shows the FA map, with brighter voxels indicating higher FA values. Image (*E*) shows the color-coded image with brightness (color intensity) again representing voxels with higher FA values and the orientation of the principal diffusion direction represented by red, green, and blue. Blue, red, and green correspond to diffusion along the inferior-superior, transverse, and anterior-posterior directions, respectfully.

centrum semiovale, and internal/external capsules.[36,43,53,60–64] These structures may be particularly vulnerable to injury due to their anatomic relationship to the skull and other structures such as the falx cerebri. Within the CC, some studies have shown the posterior part to be more vulnerable than the anterior part.[47] The CC is the most commonly identified region of abnormal FA and MD, perhaps because it is the largest WM tract in the brain and an important site of TBI pathology. For both reasons, the CC is commonly chosen as a target of analyses, a choice that may bias the findings of the literature.[10,65] For example, in one study, cognitively impaired football players in the National Football League showed decreased FA in the bilateral frontal and parietal lobes, the CC,

and the left temporal lobes compared with controls.[55] In other literature concerning MD, although some studies reported it to be normal in comparison to healthy subjects, others described it as increased in the splenium of the CC.[43,66,67] In addition to these commonly used metrics, an increased RD has been demonstrated in the genu and splenium of the CC in mTBI patients.[38] However, these findings are almost entirely based on group comparisons and do not necessarily reflect the distribution of injuries in the individual patient.[10]

Other research has been more conflicting. For example, mTBI was recently found not to be associated with WM changes in a large controlled study although previous studies showed

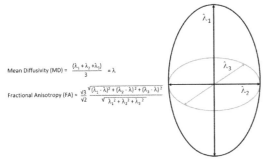

Mean Diffusivity (MD) = $\frac{(\lambda_1 + \lambda_2 + \lambda_3)}{3}$ $= \lambda$

Fractional Anisotropy (FA) = $\frac{\sqrt{3}}{\sqrt{2}} \frac{\sqrt{(\lambda_1 - \lambda)^2 + (\lambda_2 - \lambda)^2 + (\lambda_3 - \lambda)^2}}{\sqrt{\lambda_1{}^2 + \lambda_2{}^2 + \lambda_3{}^2}}$

Fig. 5. 3D ellipsoid with MD and FA formulas. Three eigenvectors define the ellipsoid axes and three associated eigenvalues (λ) define the length. The two primary metrics in DTI are MD, the total amount of diffusion in a voxel, and FA, the relative anisotropy in a voxel. AD describes diffusion along the principal axis (principal eigenvector λ1) whereas RD is an average of diffusion along its two minor axes (λ2 and λ3).

significant differences in FA for the CC, internal capsule, and external capsule.[40,67,68] These conflicting results emphasize the need for further research.

PROGNOSIS

Now that we have a general understanding of techniques and DTI metric changes observed in the WM of TBI patients, we will turn our attention toward key populations affected by TBI, focusing on mTBI, and what can be said about prognostication in the current era.

Both civilian and military populations are affected by TBI, with variables affecting injury patterns including mechanism of injury (eg, falls, motor vehicle collisions), timing from injury, and severity. Civilian sub-populations affected by TBI include children, adults, elderly, and contact

sports athletes, each with unique considerations. Although a full discussion is beyond the scope of this paper, we will focus here on pediatric, adult civilian, and adult military populations affected by TBI.

Children and Athletes

In the pediatric population, both increased and decreased FA have been associated with mTBI, similar to the results mentioned above. For example, Van Beek and colleagues studied children aged 7 to 13 years with mTBI and found an initial decrease in FA within the CC when measured within 1 month post-injury, with normalization seen at 6 to 8 months post-injury.[69] Although they also observed a persistent decreased working memory, no direct relationship with DTI metrics could be established for this outcome.[69] In other research, although Königs and colleagues did not find any mTBI biomarkers, a correlation between FA and neurocognitive functions was observed, as measured by the Full-scale Intelligence Quotient and Digit Span (a working memory and attention test).[70] However, when studying the pediatric population, the results of diffusion findings with the evolution of neurocognitive function were mixed. Another study involving a larger group of children (mean age 12.37) suffering from concussion primarily due to falls showed weak associations between parent-reported post-concussive symptoms and FA (negative) as well as MD values (positive) taken less than 2 weeks post-injury.[71]

In a study of high school football players, Lancaster and colleagues found that MD, AD, and RD measured at 24 hours and 8 days following trauma negatively correlated with Sport Concussion Assessment Tool-3 (SCAT-3) scores measured at 24 hours.[72] However, it is noteworthy

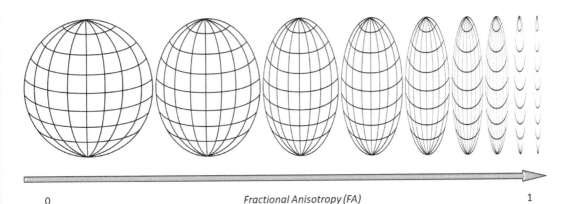

0   *Fractional Anisotropy (FA)*   1

Fig. 6. FA graphically represented, with an FA value of 0 (isoptropic diffusion) appearing as a sphere and an FA value of 1 represented by an infinite cylinder.

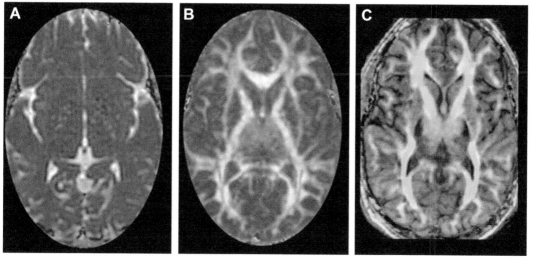

Fig. 7. Examples of MD, FA, and color-coded DTI images. Image (A) shows the mean diffusion, which is a trace of the diffusion tensor. Image (B) shows the FA map, with brighter voxels indicating higher FA values. Image (C) shows the color-coded image with brightness (color intensity) again representing voxels with higher FA values and color representing the orientation of the principal direction of diffusion. Blue, red, and green correspond to diffusion along the inferior-superior, transverse, and anterior-posterior directions, respectfully.

that mean SCAT-3 scores in the control athletes also demonstrated a slight decrease at 24 hours following sporting events, and also that no significant association was found when comparing DTI metrics with the Standardized Assessment of Concussion scores. A similar study evaluating 14- to 17-year-old athletes (mean age 15.5)

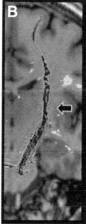

Fig. 8. Example of diffusion tensor data being used to produce a tractography map. Color-coded DTI (A) shows an example "seed site" or ROI (circle) being place over the left corticospinal tact (CST). Example of the left corticospinal tract (arrow) overlayed on a 3D FSPGR (fast spoiled gradient-echo) image (B) with the CST (blue) coursing in the superior-inferior direction.

demonstrated a positive correlation between SCAT-2 scores and MD, and an inverse correlation between SCAT-2 scores and FA, contrary to the former study.[73] These conflicting data indicate the need for additional research into the prognosticative role of DTI in sports-related injuries.

Adults

Similarly mixed results have been found in the adult mTBI population. For example, FA values have been reported by investigators as initially decreasing, with a gradual return to normal, as well as initially normal with a decrease after 12 months.[74,75] Other studies of adult mTBI patients scanned within 0 to 5 days post-trauma, including a meta-analysis of 17 studies from 2007 to 2015, have demonstrated significant decreased FA when compared with healthy controls.[74,76,77]

A meta-analysis of eight studies evaluating cognitive function following mTBI also demonstrated decreased FA with increased MD associated with both memory and attention deficits.[78] In other research, decreased FA has also been associated with prolonged post-trauma migraine recovery periods and worsened chronic cognitive impairment.[79,80] Veeramuthu and colleagues correlated acute changes in FA within the cerebellar peduncle, corona radiata, cingulum, superior longitudinal fasciculus, and splenium of the CC to changes in language and spatial function at 6 months following injury. It is worth noting

Box 1
Standard diffusion tensor imaging protocol parameters

- Prefer 3T
- Multichannel coil
- Parallel image acquisition
- 40 to 80 mT/m maximal amplitude
- 150 to 200 mT/m/ms slew rate
- b-values range from 750 to 1200 m/s
- Slice thickness of 2 mm
- Zero skip
- Matrix of 128 x 128
- 25 to 30 diffusion directions
- Voxel size 8 to 20 mm

that in this study of mTBI patients only, there was a large difference in cognitive scores when compared with healthy controls in both acute and chronic settings, despite only mild injury.

Castano-Leon and colleagues studied 118 patients with moderate to severe TBI longitudinally using both clinical metrics and DTI parameters at three spots on the CC.[81,82] In this study, they found that longitudinal FA analysis correlated with clinical recovery. However, this correlation was only at the group level, a limitation of DTI as discussed later.

A variety of other cognitive and functional outcomes in mild to severe TBI have also been correlated with DTI. For example, in patients with mTBI, severely reduced FA has been correlated with worse 3- and 6-month Glasgow Outcome Scale-Extended outcomes.[79] Additionally, in severe TBI, an increase in FA on the initial post-injury DTI has been associated with a favorable outcome, possibly secondary to axonal regrowth during later recovery.[83] Another meta-analysis involving 20 studies of adult TBI patients reported that a high FA in most areas of the brain correlated

with better cognitive outcomes, particularly memory and attention.[84]

Military

In the past two decades, many thousands of US military service members have suffered from mTBI. Although there is much overlap in the mechanisms of injury between the civilian and military populations, blast-related injuries, such as from an improvised explosive device (IED), are more common in the military setting. The shock wave generated by an IED passes through the head and can cause TBI without leaving a visible external wound. Military medical teams need to know how to best care for service members who experience these types of injuries and whether they need to be transferred to a higher level of care. Furthermore, military commanders need to know whether service members who experience blast injuries can return to duty.

Most cross-sectional imaging in the past two decades of US military conflict has been predominantly composed of CT, with some limited MR imaging capability. For the few military hospitals with MR imaging scanners, this has been primarily done using conventional techniques, without DTI capabilities. Although some military hospitals in the United States do have this capability, there is increased emphasis on providing state-o–the art diagnosis and prognosis downrange to the point of initial care. In addition to applying lessons learned from civilian populations, DTI is one of many techniques that are actively being explored to assist in providing state-of-the-art diagnosis and prognosis to military service members in the theater.

LIMITATIONS

Despite some promising advances, there are important limitations that must be understood when interpreting DTI, several of which will be discussed here. We have broadly grouped these limitations into technical, lack of specificity, and study heterogeneity (Fig. 10).

Technical

Although a full discussion of technical limitations of DTI is outside the scope of this review, and has been previously described in greater detail, a few require specific mention.[31]

Perhaps most notably is the issue of crossing fibers. The diffusion tensor model assumes that there is a single ellipsoid with all axons traveling in the same direction within each imaging voxel. Although this may be time efficient, many fiber

Timing   Severity   Location

Fig. 9. Primary factors affecting the DTI findings in TBI including time between injury onset and imaging, severity of the injury, and location of the injury within the brain.

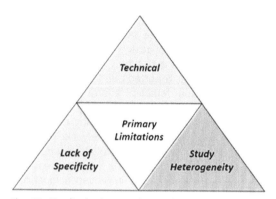

Fig. 10. Key limitations in the application of DTI in TBI include technical factors, lack of specificity, and study heterogeneity.

tracts cross several other tracts before reaching their final destination, and DTI lacks the ability to assess crossing fiber tracts within a voxel.[85–88] Regions where this is most evident include the pons, where the corticospinal tract (CST) and middle cerebellar peduncle cross, and the centrum semiovale, where the CST crosses the CC and the superior longitudinal fasciculus.[89] These locations of crossing fibers show a loss of anisotropy and reduced FA value, thereby, appearing dark on gray scale and color FA maps (Fig. 11). This can be a major limitation and more sophisticated techniques will be required to resolve this issue, particularly for smaller tracts. Advanced techniques, such as diffusion kurtosis imaging (DKI), discussed later, are seeking to overcome this limitation.[24,25,90–99]

Another important technical limitation is motion artifact. DTI pulse sequences can take several minutes to acquire, particularly when whole brain coverage is desired. Longer scan times produce a greater potential for motion. Movement artifacts can alter both FA and MD values, potentially leading to spurious conclusions.[100,101] Accelerated protocols such as reducing echo time (TE), parallel imaging, and multiband imaging can reduce scan times threefold to fivefold and help mitigate the effects of motion.[100,102–104]

Attention should also be paid to acquisition technique, as differences with technique (both within and between scanners) can alter DTI interpretation and FA values, for which phantoms have been proposed to address this issue. Other potential limitations include the selection of FA and angular thresholds, as well as ROI selection, which can introduce bias in the results.[31]

Lack of Specificity

Another important limitation of DTI is its relative lack of specificity, for reasons described above and as follows.

There is still active debate on the relationship of mTBI with diffusivity metrics, demonstrated through conflicting results for FA, MD, RD, and AD. Some studies show increased FA (suggested due to axial gliosis, selective cross-fiber degeneration), and others show decreased FA (suggested due to direct axonal injury, edema). This does not come as a surprise, given that all existing diffusion correlations in mTBI, including neurite orientation

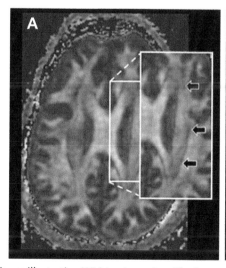

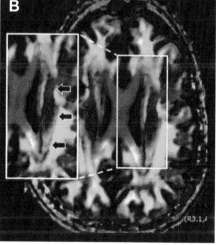

Fig. 11. Figure illustrating WM tract crossing. The image on the left (A) shows the FA map with zoomed-in image depicting a dark band (arrows) in the corona radiata where the cortical spinal tracts and superior longitudinal fasciculus intersect. The dark band occurs because the tensor model cannot distinguish low FA within a WM fiber tract from crossing fibers. Similar findings are shown on the right (B) color image where the blue corticospinal tracts and green superior longitudinal fasciculus tracts intersect, creating a dark line (arrows).

dispersion and density imaging (NODDI), are tenuous, and slight unknown confounders in study population or variable selection may swing the correlation in a completely different direction.[105,106] With diffusion metrics uniformly differing by just a few percentage points, despite the excellent intraobserver and interobserver reliability and excellent intrascanner and interscanner reproducibility, the margins of error introduced by these factors and others can be sufficient to drown out any effect from mTBI.[107,108]

Furthermore, although research studies have demonstrated that DTI is sensitive to TBI at the group level, there is insufficient evidence to suggest that DTI can be used to diagnose TBI on the individual patient level for a variety of reasons.[28,59,109–111] For example, many other diseases, including those external to the axon such as vasogenic edema, can have altered anisotropy and FA values, thereby, confounding interpretation in individual patients.[112] These causes include but are not limited to vascular conditions (eg, ischemia/infarction), inflammation/demyelination (eg, multiple sclerosis), malformation (eg, GM heterotopias, cortical dysplasias), neurodegenerative disease (eg, Alzheimer, Parkinson's, amyotrophic lateral sclerosis), psychiatric disease (eg, bipolar disorder, substance abuse), tumor (eg, mass and surrounding signal abnormality), and epilepsy as potential etiologies (Fig. 12).[31] Furthermore, some studies have failed to eliminate the potential confound of morbidity due to the experience of trauma itself, rather than adverse outcomes specifically due to TBI.[10] FA values also vary as patients age and studies must control for this.[71] FA values must therefore be interpreted with caution and in the full clinical context.

Another contributor to the lack of specificity is the lack of a normative imaging database that is stratified by age, sex, and comorbidities, which could provide a clear understanding of normal variations across populations and to which patients with TBI could be compared.[35] Efforts have been made to construct such as database as will be discussed later.

Study Heterogeneity

Another major limitation has been the heterogenous nature of previous studies which makes it difficult to draw conclusions.[113] Studies have differed substantially in terms of patient populations, comorbidities, mechanism, location of injury, timing, imaging protocols, brain regions examined, analysis type, measurement technique (eg, ROI selection), treatment, and follow-up.[10] For most research studies, trauma patients are lumped into one group, which may mask differences based on these factors.[10] Many studies use a cross-sectional design and do not compare individual changes over time.[10] Furthermore, mild TBI is likely under-reported due to mild symptoms that may escape detection and/or due to fear of being removed from work or play (eg, military, athletes, pilots). Heterogeneity in study design and how TBI presents in humans is likely a key contributor as to why some neuroprotective strategies which have positive outcomes in animal research have failed to translate to improved clinical outcomes in clinical TBI trials.[114–119]

FUTURE DIRECTIONS

Future directions for evaluating TBI include advanced techniques, developing a normative database, continued research, and machine learning approaches (Fig. 13).

Advanced Techniques

Several technical advances are currently being investigated to address some of the shortcomings not addressed with modern DTI. Complete discussions about these methods are outside the scope of this article but have been previously reviewed.[28,31,89] Within conventional DTI, researchers have been looking beyond traditional metrics such as FA and MD values at the regional or whole brain level, and exploring other metrics such as AD and RD as potentially more specific markers of TBI.[120]

Additionally, as previously mentioned, one of the main limitations of DTI is its inability to assess fiber tracts crossing within a voxel.[28,85–88] Thus, there is considerable research in the development of newer DTI techniques, also referred to as high-level tractography, including other model-based techniques, such as DKI and NODDI, as well as model-free techniques, such as Diffusion Spectrum Imaging (DSI) to improve visualization of tracts within a voxel, particularly with crossing fibers (Fig. 14).[24,25,90–99,121] These techniques use various algorithms, but ultimately result in a greater sampling of q-space (the three-dimensional space defined by diffusion gradients in the x, y, and z planes) and improved modeling of neural connections (Fig. 15). A main drawback, however, is the greater computing complexity and increased time of imaging acquisition (which can lead to more motion), although accelerated protocols are possible in some instances.[120,122]

There is also increasing emphasis on exploring more complex patterns of diffusion that more closely resemble the biological tissue. As previously mentioned, DTI data are a simplified

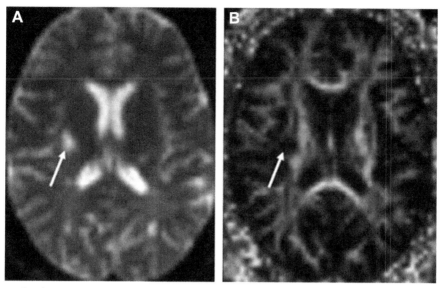

Fig. 12. Example of a young woman with multiple sclerosis and altered FA values. (*A*) Transverse b0 image shows a focus of signal abnormality (*arrow*) in the right corona radiata. (*B*) Transverse FA map of the lesion (*arrow*) showing decreased anisotropy. Many diseases, including multiple sclerosis, can have altered anisotropy and thereby confound interpretation in patients who have experienced a TBI. (*From* Nucifora PG, Verma R, Lee SK, Melhem ER. Diffusion-tensor MR imaging and tractography: exploring brain microstructure and connectivity. Radiology. Nov 2007;245(2):367-84; with permission.)

Gaussian-based mathematic model describing the normative distribution of a given population conforming to a bell curve. However, biological tissues are a highly heterogeneous media with various compartments and barriers causing the diffusion of water molecules to deviate considerably from this pattern.[120] Therefore, although

useful for its simplicity, this has inherent inaccuracies. DKI is a non-Gaussian model attempting to account for this variation and improve accuracy, with the term kurtosis (K) used to capture the deviation for the Gaussian distribution (Fig. 16).[120] Parameters such as mean kurtosis (MK), radial kurtosis (RK), and axial kurtosis (AK) are being investigated, as well as data that may complement DTI metrics such as MK-MD mismatch to increase specificity.[91] For example, reduced MK within the thalamus in patients with mild TBI was associated with cognitive impairment on 1-year follow-up, suggesting this may serve as an early predictor of brain damage.[123] More studies are required to further validate the data and link DKI changes to pathologic findings.[124] Through these technical advances, more specific diagnoses can be made and potentially coupled with more specific treatments.

Normative Database

As previously mentioned, one major barrier to implementing these technical advances in TBI is the lack of a normative database. At the 2014 TBI workshop in Montreal, Canada, the American Society of Neuroradiology, American College of Radiology, Head Injury Institute, and American Society for Functional Neuroradiology , TBI experts discussed the formation of the ideal database, normal control subject, and standardizing clinical

Advanced Techniques

Normative Database

Continued Research

Machine Learning

Fig. 13. Future directions for evaluating TBI include advanced techniques, developing a normative database, continued research, and machine learning approaches.

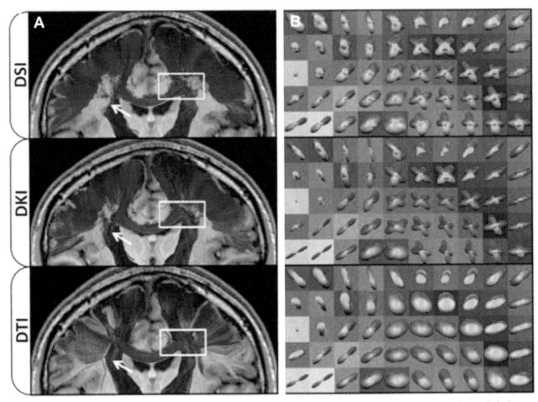

Fig. 14. –Example of different advanced tractography techniques on displaying WM tracts. Column (*A*) shows a coronal cross-section through the fiber tracts identified with DSI, DKI, and DTI, overlaid on a 3D T1-weighted image for anatomic reference. The colors represent the predominant tract orientation where red represents an overall left-right orientation, blue represents an overall inferior-superior orientation, and green represents an overall anterior-posterior orientation. DSI and DKI are similar with respect to the color (overall trajectory) and distribution of fibers identified. However, DSI seems to be the most sensitive technique for detecting some fibers (*white arrows*). Column (*B*) shows a select portion of the fibers from column A (*white box*) with a high degree of fiber crossing (corpus callosum, corona radiata, superior longitudinal fasciculus, and cingulum bundle) using the same coloring scheme for orientation. DTI cannot detect crossing fibers causing fibers to prematurely terminate (or meld) anatomically distinct tracts whereas DSI and DKI are better able to resolve this. (*From* Glenn GR, Kuo LW, Chao YP, Lee CY, Helpern JA, Jensen JH. Mapping the Orientation of White Matter Fiber Bundles: A Comparative Study of Diffusion Tensor Imaging, Diffusional Kurtosis Imaging, and Diffusion Spectrum Imaging. *AJNR Am J Neuroradiol*. Jul 2016;37(7):1216-22.)

and research neuroimaging protocols.[35] Many existing platforms exist and should be used by the TBI community to create such a database.[35] A skilled neuroradiologist should review all the imaging data before deposition of the data in the normative database, and the imaging data should also be reviewed once within the database by an independent qualified team.[35] However, constructing a large comprehensive normative database has several challenges, such as defining what is normal, distinguishing acute from chronic abnormalities in patients with pre-existing conditions, creating protocols that work with multiple vendors (across platforms and institutions), as well as creating data-sharing repositories to apply informatics tools.[35] Nonetheless, such a database

is necessary to allow for advances in traditional and machine learning research.

Research

As previously mentioned, the literature demonstrates an overall high between-study heterogeneity with variable clinical heterogeneity including patient population, comorbidities, timing of TBI, mechanism of injury, site of injury, and methodological heterogeneities with regard to imaging protocol, length of follow-up, and modes of assessment. Such heterogeneity in TBI poses a challenge in identifying an effective treatment and is perhaps one reason why promising animal research has failed to translate into improved clinical outcomes in clinical TBI trials.[113–117]

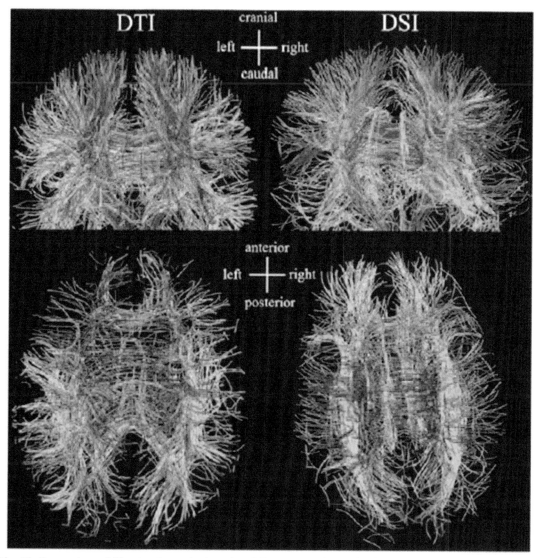

Fig. 15. Comparison of fiber tractography based on DTI versus DSI in two healthy volunteers. Coronal (*top row*) and axial (*bottom row*) show that fiber crossing on DSI is better resolved and fibers from different tracts are more clearly separated because DSI provides higher angular resolution. This is most notable with the greater number of red tracts (decussating callosal fibers) and a more uniform distribution of fibers projecting into the frontal lobe on DSI. (*From* Hagmann P, Jonasson L, Maeder P, Thiran JP, Wedeen VJ, Meuli R. Understanding diffusion MR imaging techniques: from scalar diffusion-weighted imaging to diffusion tensor imaging and beyond. Radiographics. Oct 2006;26 Suppl 1:S205-23; with permission.)

Therefore, using a normative database, future studies will need to account for this heterogeneity looking at DTI changes with different severities and chronicity, as well as longitudinal studies looking at changes that evolve. Most studies include subacute TBI due to ease of enrollment and chronic patients are often lost to follow-up.[10] Techniques should be standardized and performed with both the regional and whole brain analysis, in addition to the advanced techniques described earlier to draw meaningful conclusions.[10] Outcome measures will also need to be explicitly defined and incorporated into statistical models.[10]

Machine Learning

Machine learning, specifically deep learning, algorithms have been very successful in a wide range of applications from computer vision to imaging in health care. The increasing role of machine learning and deep learning in high-risk

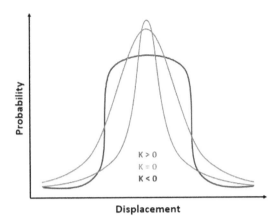

Fig. 16. Diffusion kurtosis graph showing how a diffusion displacement probability distribution varies in appearance with different values of kurtosis (K). A Gaussian distribution (ie, bell curve) is represented by a K value of "0" whereas deviation from the Gaussian distribution in represented by a non-zero number.

applications, such as health care, has been demonstrated by obtaining human-level or even better than human-level performances. Neuroimaging and clinical applications of neuroimaging have also greatly benefited from recent advances in deep learning technologies, with newly developed predictors and classifiers using various MR imaging sequences (eg, DWI, functional MR imaging) for common neurologic diseases including Alzheimer's disease, Parkinson's, and epilepsy. Deep learning-based predictive systems may aid in the diagnosis and prognosis of such diseases, as well as advance our knowledge about their underlying biological mechanisms by using imaging and non-imaging data in a way that was not previously possible.

However, despite tremendous findings in neuroimaging studies with deep learning, deep learning-based TBI studies are limited to date. Existing studies used simple machine learning or earlier versions of deep learning algorithms with multimodal imaging data including DTI with a limited number of patients.[125,126] Even with these limitations, there are some promising results that TBI can be explored better with machine learning algorithms.[122,127–130] Research with artificial intelligence (AI) has made tremendous progress over the past decade. Tasks such as segmentation, localization of pathologies, lateralization, diagnosis, and prognosis have substantially improved. The AI-powered images and signals have reached human-level performance or better in many applications, including biomedical imaging. This is mainly due to the strengths of AI algorithms to discover potential patterns and relations from any data in general, and specifically neuroimaging data. Hence, the future of neuroimaging and its clinical applications can be enhanced through the integration of such algorithms.

SUMMARY

DTI is a technique that has shown promising, albeit sometimes conflicting, results in diagnosing TBI-related injuries and providing prognostic information. Like all techniques, however, it is not without limitations, most notably of which are the inherently subtle changes in diffusion metrics with TBI, as well as the inability to resolve crossing WM tract fibers. Advanced imaging and image analysis techniques, coupled with the development of a normative database to conduct both traditional and machine learning-based research, will be needed to translate this technique from the lab to the clinic and help guide tomorrow's treatments.

CLINICS CARE POINTS

- DTI generally shows low FA and high MD values in patients with TBI-related injury. However, many diseases can also show altered FA and MD values. Results should therefore be interpreted with caution and in the full clinical context.

- A key limitation of DTI is its inability to resolve crossing WM tract fibers within a voxel. Advanced techniques, such as DKI, can better resolve this at the expense of increased imaging time and more involved computing.

- Although research shows a general trend toward low FA values in TBI patients, this can only be said at the group level and exact cutoffs differentiating normal versus abnormal have not yet been established to allow these data to be applied to individual patients. Future research will better clarify this.

DISCLOSURE

M. Grant: None. J. Liu: None. M. Wintermark: None. U. Bagci: None. D. Douglas: None. M. Grant and D. Douglas: The views expressed are those of the author(s) and do not reflect the official policy of the Department of the Army, the Department of the Air Force, the Department of Defense, or the US Government.

REFERENCES

1. Marr AL, Coronado VG. Central nervous system injury surveillance data submission standards—2002. Atlanta, GA: Centers for Disease Control and Prevention, National Center for Injury Prevention and Control; 2004.
2. Faul M, National Center for Injury Prevention and Control (U.S.). Traumatic brain injury in the United States : emergency department visits, hospitalizations, and deaths, 2002-2006.1 online resource (vii, 70 pages). Available at: http://purl.fdlp.gov/GPO/gpo41911. Accessed June 4, 2022.
3. Marin JR, Weaver MD, Yealy DM, et al. Trends in visits for traumatic brain injury to emergency departments in the United States. JAMA 2014; 311(18):1917–9.
4. Centers for Disease C Prevention. Nonfatal traumatic brain injuries related to sports and recreation activities among persons aged </=19 years–United States, 2001-2009. MMWR Morbidity and mortality weekly report 2011;60(39):1337–42.
5. Centers for Disease C. Prevention. Traumatic Brain Injury & Concussion. 2021. Available at: https://www.cdc.gov/traumaticbraininjury/. Accessed September 14, 2021.
6. Corrigan JD, Selassie AW, Orman JA. The epidemiology of traumatic brain injury. Journal of head trauma rehabilitation 2010;25(2):72–80.
7. Strauss S, Hulkower M, Gulko E, et al. Current Clinical Applications and Future Potential of Diffusion Tensor Imaging in Traumatic Brain Injury. Top Magn Reson Imaging 2015;24(6): 353–62.
8. Miller GF, DePadilla L, Xu L. Costs of Nonfatal Traumatic Brain Injury in the United States, 2016. Med Care 2021;59(5):451–5.
9. Bass E, Golding H, United States. Congressional Budget Office. *The Veterans Health Administration's treatment of PTSD and traumatic brain injury among recent combat veterans.* Congress of the United States. Washington, DC: Congressional Budget Office; 2012. p. 1. online resource (ix, 39 p.) Available at: http://purl.fdlp.gov/GPO/gpo18872.
10. Hulkower MB, Poliak DB, Rosenbaum SB, et al. A decade of DTI in traumatic brain injury: 10 years and 100 articles later. AJNR Am J Neuroradiol 2013;34(11):2064–74.
11. Teasdale G, Jennett B. Assessment of coma and impaired consciousness: a practical scale. Lancet 1974;304(7872):81–4.
12. Smith LGF, Milliron E, Ho ML, et al. Advanced neuroimaging in traumatic brain injury: an overview. Neurosurg Focus 2019;47(6):E17.
13. McCrory P, Meeuwisse W, Johnston K, et al. Consensus statement on concussion in sport: the 3rd International Conference on Concussion in Sport held in Zurich, November 2008. Journal of athletic training 2009;44(4):434–48.
14. Golby AJ, Kindlmann G, Norton I, et al. Interactive diffusion tensor tractography visualization for neurosurgical planning. Neurosurgery 2011;68(2): 496–505.
15. Gong G, He Y, Concha L, et al. Mapping anatomical connectivity patterns of human cerebral cortex using in vivo diffusion tensor imaging tractography. Cerebral cortex 2009;19(3):524–36.
16. Johansen-Berg H. Behavioural relevance of variation in white matter microstructure. Curr Opin Neurol 2010;23(4):351–8.
17. Basser PJ, Jones DK. Diffusion-tensor MRI: theory, experimental design and data analysis - a technical review. NMR in biomedicine 2002;15(7–8): 456–67.
18. Mori S. Introduction to diffusion tensor imaging. Amsterdam, Netherlands: Elsiever; 2007.
19. Le Bihan D. Looking into the functional architecture of the brain with diffusion MRI. Nat Rev Neurosci 2003;4(6):469–80.
20. Behrens TJ-B,H. Diffusion MRI: from quantitative measurements to in vivo neuroanatomy. Cambridge, Massachusetts: Academic Press; 2009.
21. Le Bihan D, Mangin JF, Poupon C, et al. Diffusion tensor imaging: concepts and applications. J Magn Reson Imag 2001;13(4):534–46.
22. Mori S, Zhang J. Principles of diffusion tensor imaging and its applications to basic neuroscience research. Neuron 2006;51(5):527–39.
23. Beaulieu C. The basis of anisotropic water diffusion in the nervous system - a technical review. NMR in biomedicine 2002;15(7–8):435–55.
24. Teipel SJ, Stahl R, Dietrich O, et al. Multivariate network analysis of fiber tract integrity in Alzheimer's disease. Neuroimage 2007;34(3):985–95.
25. Jones DK, Cercignani M. Twenty-five pitfalls in the analysis of diffusion MRI data. NMR in biomedicine 2010;23(7):803–20.
26. Basser PJ. New histological and physiological stains derived from diffusion-tensor MR images. Ann N Y Acad Sci 1997;820:123–38.
27. Basser PJ, Mattiello J, LeBihan D. Estimation of the effective self-diffusion tensor from the NMR spin echo. Journal of magnetic resonance Series B 1994;103(3):247–54.
28. Douglas DB, Iv M, Douglas PK, et al. Diffusion Tensor Imaging of TBI: Potentials and Challenges. Top Magn Reson Imaging 2015;24(5):241–51.
29. Skare S, Hedehus M, Moseley ME, et al. Condition number as a measure of noise performance of diffusion tensor data acquisition schemes with MRI. Journal of magnetic resonance 2000;147(2): 340–52.
30. Kaplan PE. Encyclopedia of clinical neuropsychology. New York: Springer; 2011. p. 1074.

31. Nucifora PG, Verma R, Lee SK, et al. Diffusion-tensor MR imaging and tractography: exploring brain microstructure and connectivity. Radiology 2007;245(2):367–84.

32. Mandl RC, Schnack HG, Zwiers MP, et al. Functional diffusion tensor imaging at 3 Tesla. Front Hum Neurosci 2013;7:817.

33. Mori S, Setsuwakana, Nagae-Poetscher LM, et al. MRI atlas of human white matter. Amsterdam, Netherlands: Elsevier; 2005.

34. Jones DK, Leemans A. Diffusion tensor imaging. Methods Mol Biol 2011;711:127–44.

35. Wintermark M, Coombs L, Druzgal TJ, et al. Traumatic brain injury imaging research roadmap. AJNR Am J Neuroradiol 2015;36(3):E12–23.

36. Bazarian JJ, Zhong J, Blyth B, et al. Diffusion tensor imaging detects clinically important axonal damage after mild traumatic brain injury: a pilot study. J Neurotrauma 2007;24(9):1447–59.

37. Wilde EA, McCauley SR, Hunter JV, et al. Diffusion tensor imaging of acute mild traumatic brain injury in adolescents. Neurology 2008;70(12):948–55.

38. Delouche A, Attyé A, Heck O, et al. Diffusion MRI: Pitfalls, literature review and future directions of research in mild traumatic brain injury. Eur J Radiol 2016;85(1):25–30.

39. Wilde EA, Ramos MA, Yallampalli R, et al. Diffusion tensor imaging of the cingulum bundle in children after traumatic brain injury. Dev Neuropsychol 2010;35(3):333–51.

40. Arfanakis K, Haughton VM, Carew JD, et al. Diffusion tensor MR imaging in diffuse axonal injury. AJNR Am J Neuroradiol 2002;23(5):794–802.

41. Kumar R, Gupta RK, Husain M, et al. Comparative evaluation of corpus callosum DTI metrics in acute mild and moderate traumatic brain injury: its correlation with neuropsychometric tests. Brain Inj 2009; 23(7):675–85.

42. Newcombe VF, Williams GB, Nortje J, et al. Concordant biology underlies discordant imaging findings: diffusivity behaves differently in grey and white matter post acute neurotrauma. Acta Neurochir Suppl 2008;102:247–51.

43. Miles L, Grossman RI, Johnson G, et al. Short-term DTI predictors of cognitive dysfunction in mild traumatic brain injury. Brain Inj 2008;22(2):115–22.

44. Newcombe VF, Williams GB, Nortje J, et al. Analysis of acute traumatic axonal injury using diffusion tensor imaging. Br J Neurosurg 2007;21(4):340–8.

45. Wozniak JR, Lim KO. Advances in white matter imaging: a review of in vivo magnetic resonance methodologies and their applicability to the study of development and aging. Neurosci Biobehav Rev 2006;30(6):762–74.

46. Wozniak JR, Krach L, Ward E, et al. Neurocognitive and neuroimaging correlates of pediatric traumatic brain injury: a diffusion tensor imaging (DTI) study. Arch Clin Neuropsychol 2007;22(5):555–68.

47. Aoki Y, Inokuchi R, Gunshin M, et al. Diffusion tensor imaging studies of mild traumatic brain injury: a meta-analysis. J Neurol Neurosurg Psychiatr 2012;83(9):870–6.

48. Brandstack N, Kurki T, Tenovuo O. Quantitative diffusion-tensor tractography of long association tracts in patients with traumatic brain injury without associated findings at routine MR imaging. Radiology 2013;267(1):231–9.

49. Davenport ND, Lim KO, Armstrong MT, et al. Diffuse and spatially variable white matter disruptions are associated with blast-related mild traumatic brain injury. Neuroimage 2012;59(3): 2017–24.

50. Mayer AR, Ling JM, Yang Z, et al. Diffusion abnormalities in pediatric mild traumatic brain injury. J Neurosci 2012;32(50):17961–9.

51. Ling JM, Pena A, Yeo RA, et al. Biomarkers of increased diffusion anisotropy in semi-acute mild traumatic brain injury: a longitudinal perspective. Brain 2012;135(Pt 4):1281–92.

52. Chu Z, Wilde EA, Hunter JV, et al. Voxel-based analysis of diffusion tensor imaging in mild traumatic brain injury in adolescents. AJNR Am J Neuroradiol 2010;31(2):340–6.

53. Mayer AR, Ling J, Mannell MV, et al. A prospective diffusion tensor imaging study in mild traumatic brain injury. Neurology 2010;74(8):643–50.

54. Mac Donald CL, Johnson AM, Cooper D, et al. Detection of blast-related traumatic brain injury in U.S. military personnel. N Engl J Med 2011; 364(22):2091–100.

55. Hart J Jr, Kraut MA, Womack KB, et al. Neuroimaging of cognitive dysfunction and depression in aging retired National Football League players: a cross-sectional study. JAMA neurology 2013; 70(3):326–35.

56. Kim N, Branch CA, Kim M, et al. Whole brain approaches for identification of microstructural abnormalities in individual patients: comparison of techniques applied to mild traumatic brain injury. PLoS One 2013;8(3):e59382.

57. Lipton ML, Gulko E, Zimmerman ME, et al. Diffusion-tensor imaging implicates prefrontal axonal injury in executive function impairment following very mild traumatic brain injury. Radiology 2009; 252(3):816–24.

58. Wallace EJ, Mathias JL, Ward L. Diffusion tensor imaging changes following mild, moderate and severe adult traumatic brain injury: a meta-analysis. Brain Imaging Behav 2018;12(6):1607–21.

59. Wintermark M, Sanelli PC, Anzai Y, et al. Imaging evidence and recommendations for traumatic brain injury: advanced neuro- and neurovascular

imaging techniques. AJNR Am J Neuroradiol 2015; 36(2):E1–11.

60. Bazarian JJ, Donnelly K, Peterson DR, et al. The relation between posttraumatic stress disorder and mild traumatic brain injury acquired during Operations Enduring Freedom and Iraqi Freedom. J Head Trauma Rehabil 2013;28(1):1–12.

61. Henry LC, Tremblay J, Tremblay S, et al. Acute and chronic changes in diffusivity measures after sports concussion. J Neurotrauma 2011;28(10): 2049–59.

62. Rutgers DR, Fillard P, Paradot G, et al. Diffusion tensor imaging characteristics of the corpus callosum in mild, moderate, and severe traumatic brain injury. AJNR Am J Neuroradiol 2008;29(9):1730–5.

63. Nakayama N, Okumura A, Shinoda J, et al. Evidence for white matter disruption in traumatic brain injury without macroscopic lesions. J Neurol Neurosurg Psychiatr 2006;77(7):850–5.

64. Levin HS, Wilde EA, Chu Z, et al. Diffusion tensor imaging in relation to cognitive and functional outcome of traumatic brain injury in children. J Head Trauma Rehabil 2008;23(4):197–208.

65. Hernandez F, Giordano C, Goubran M, et al. Lateral impacts correlate with falx cerebri displacement and corpus callosum trauma in sports-related concussions. Biomech Model Mechanobiol 2019; 18(3):631–49.

66. Tuch DS, Reese TG, Wiegell MR, et al. High angular resolution diffusion imaging reveals intravoxel white matter fiber heterogeneity. Magn Reson Med 2002;48(4):577–82.

67. Inglese M, Makani S, Johnson G, et al. Diffuse axonal injury in mild traumatic brain injury: a diffusion tensor imaging study. J Neurosurg 2005; 103(2):298–303.

68. Ilvesmäki T, Luoto TM, Hakulinen U, et al. Acute mild traumatic brain injury is not associated with white matter change on diffusion tensor imaging. Brain 2014;137(Pt 7):1876–82.

69. Van Beek L, Vanderauwera J, Ghesquiere P, et al. Longitudinal changes in mathematical abilities and white matter following paediatric mild traumatic brain injury. Brain Inj 2015;29(13–14): 1701–10.

70. Konigs M, Pouwels PJ, Ernest van Heurn LW, et al. Relevance of neuroimaging for neurocognitive and behavioral outcome after pediatric traumatic brain injury. Brain Imaging Behav 2018;12(1):29–43.

71. Ware AL, Shukla A, Goodrich-Hunsaker NJ, et al. Post-acute white matter microstructure predicts post-acute and chronic post-concussive symptom severity following mild traumatic brain injury in children. Neuroimage Clin 2020;25:102106.

72. Lancaster MA, Olson DV, McCrea MA, et al. Acute white matter changes following sport-related concussion: A serial diffusion tensor and diffusion kurtosis tensor imaging study. Hum Brain Mapp 2016;37(11):3821–34.

73. Virji-Babul N, Borich MR, Makan N, et al. Diffusion tensor imaging of sports-related concussion in adolescents. Pediatr Neurol 2013;48(1):24–9.

74. Yin B, Li DD, Huang H, et al. Longitudinal Changes in Diffusion Tensor Imaging Following Mild Traumatic Brain Injury and Correlation With Outcome. Front Neural Circuits 2019;13:28.

75. Studerus-Germann AM, Gautschi OP, Bontempi P, et al. Central nervous system microbleeds in the acute phase are associated with structural integrity by DTI one year after mild traumatic brain injury: A longitudinal study. Neurol Neurochir Pol 2018; 52(6):710–9.

76. Veeramuthu V, Narayanan V, Kuo TL, et al. Diffusion Tensor Imaging Parameters in Mild Traumatic Brain Injury and Its Correlation with Early Neuropsychological Impairment: A Longitudinal Study. J Neurotrauma 2015;32(19):1497–509.

77. Aoki Y, Inokuchi R. A voxel-based meta-analysis of diffusion tensor imaging in mild traumatic brain injury. Neurosci Biobehav Rev 2016;66:119–26.

78. Oehr L, Anderson J. Diffusion-Tensor Imaging Findings and Cognitive Function Following Hospitalized Mixed-Mechanism Mild Traumatic Brain Injury: A Systematic Review and Meta-Analysis. Arch Phys Med Rehabil 2017;98(11):2308–19.

79. Yuh EL, Cooper SR, Mukherjee P, et al. Diffusion tensor imaging for outcome prediction in mild traumatic brain injury: a TRACK-TBI study. J Neurotrauma 2014;31(17):1457–77.

80. Alhilali LM, Delic J, Fakhran S. Differences in Callosal and Forniceal Diffusion between Patients with and without Postconcussive Migraine. AJNR Am J Neuroradiol 2017;38(4):691–5.

81. Castaño-Leon AM, Cicuendez M, Navarro-Main B, et al. Sixto Obrador SENEC prize 2019: Utility of diffusion tensor imaging as a prognostic tool in moderate to severe traumatic brain injury. Part I. Analysis of DTI metrics performed during the early subacute stage. Neurocirugia (Astur : Engl Ed) 2020;31(3):132–45. Premio Sixto Obrador SENEC 2019: el uso de la secuencia tensor de difusión como herramienta pronóstica en los pacientes con traumatismo craneoencefálico grave y moderado. Parte I. Análisis de las características del tensor de difusión realizado durante la fase subaguda precoz.

82. Castaño-Leon AM, Cicuendez M, Navarro-Main B, et al. SIXTO OBRADOR SENEC PRIZE 2019: Utility of diffusion tensor imaging as a prognostic tool in moderate to severe traumatic brain injury. Part II: Longitudinal analysis of DTI metrics and its association with patient's outcome. Neurocirugia (Astur : Engl Ed) 2020;31(5):231–48. PREMIO SIXTO OBRADOR SENEC 2019: El uso de la secuencia

Tensor de difusión como herramienta pronóstica en los pacientes con traumatismo craneoencefálico grave y moderado. Parte II: Análisis longitudinal de las características del Tensor de difusión y su relación con la evolución de los pacientes.

83. Sidaros A, Engberg AW, Sidaros K, et al. Diffusion tensor imaging during recovery from severe traumatic brain injury and relation to clinical outcome: a longitudinal study. Brain 2008;131(Pt 2):559–72.

84. Wallace EJ, Mathias JL, Ward L. The relationship between diffusion tensor imaging findings and cognitive outcomes following adult traumatic brain injury: A meta-analysis. Neurosci Biobehav Rev 2018;92:93–103.

85. Wheeler-Kingshott CA, Cercignani M. About "axial" and "radial" diffusivities. Magn Reson Med 2009; 61(5):1255–60.

86. DK J. Challenges and limitations of quantifying brain connectivity in vivo with diffusion MRI. Imag Med 2010;2:341–55.

87. Jeurissen B, Leemans A, Tournier JD, et al. Investigating the prevalence of complex fiber configurations in white matter tissue with diffusion magnetic resonance imaging. Hum Brain Mapp 2013;34(11):2747–66.

88. Behrens TE, Berg HJ, Jbabdi S, et al. Probabilistic diffusion tractography with multiple fibre orientations: What can we gain? Neuroimage 2007;34(1): 144–55.

89. Hagmann P, Jonasson L, Maeder P, et al. Understanding diffusion MR imaging techniques: from scalar diffusion-weighted imaging to diffusion tensor imaging and beyond. Radiographics 2006; 26(Suppl 1):S205–23.

90. Zhang H, Schneider T, Wheeler-Kingshott CA, et al. NODDI: practical in vivo neurite orientation dispersion and density imaging of the human brain. Neuroimage 2012;61(4):1000–16.

91. DeCarlo LT. On the Meaning and Use of Kurtosis. Psychol Methods 1997;2(3):292–307.

92. Lazar M, Jensen JH, Xuan L, et al. Estimation of the orientation distribution function from diffusional kurtosis imaging. Magn Reson Med 2008;60(4): 774–81.

93. Umesh Rudrapatna S, Wieloch T, Beirup K, et al. Can diffusion kurtosis imaging improve the sensitivity and specificity of detecting microstructural alterations in brain tissue chronically after experimental stroke? Comparisons with diffusion tensor imaging and histology. Neuroimage 2014; 97:363–73.

94. Van AT, Granziera C, Bammer R. An introduction to model-independent diffusion magnetic resonance imaging. Top Magn Reson Imaging 2010;21(6): 339–54.

95. Jones DK, Horsfield MA, Simmons A. Optimal strategies for measuring diffusion in anisotropic systems by magnetic resonance imaging. Magn Reson Med 1999;42(3):515–25.

96. Wedeen VJ, Hagmann P, Tseng WY, et al. Mapping complex tissue architecture with diffusion spectrum magnetic resonance imaging. Magn Reson Med 2005;54(6):1377–86.

97. Tian L, Yan H, Zhang D. [Diffusion spectrum magnetic resonance imaging]. Beijing Da Xue Xue Bao Yi Xue Ban 2009;41(6):716–20.

98. Kuo LW, Chen JH, Wedeen VJ, et al. Optimization of diffusion spectrum imaging and q-ball imaging on clinical MRI system. Neuroimage 2008;41(1): 7–18.

99. G. K. Application Guide EP2D DSI Work-in-Progress Package for Diffusion Spectrum Imaging in Siemens. 2008.

100. Moeller S, Yacoub E, Olman CA, et al. Multiband multislice GE-EPI at 7 tesla, with 16-fold acceleration using partial parallel imaging with application to high spatial and temporal whole-brain fMRI. Magn Reson Med 2010;63(5):1144–53.

101. Yendiki A, Koldewyn K, Kakunoori S, et al. Spurious group differences due to head motion in a diffusion MRI study. Neuroimage 2013;88C:79–90.

102. Bammer R, Auer M, Keeling SL, et al. Diffusion tensor imaging using single-shot SENSE-EPI. Magn Reson Med 2002;48(1):128–36.

103. Feinberg DA, Setsompop K. Ultra-fast MRI of the human brain with simultaneous multi-slice imaging. Journal of magnetic resonance 2013;229:90–100.

104. Kong XZ. Association between in-scanner head motion with cerebral white matter microstructure: a multiband diffusion-weighted MRI study. PeerJ 2014;2:e366.

105. Karlsen RH, Einarsen C, Moe HK, et al. Diffusion kurtosis imaging in mild traumatic brain injury and postconcussional syndrome. J Neurosci Res 2019;97(5):568–81.

106. Oehr LE, Yang JY, Chen J, et al. Investigating White Matter Tract Microstructural Changes at Six-Twelve Weeks following Mild Traumatic Brain Injury: A Combined Diffusion Tensor Imaging and Neurite Orientation Dispersion and Density Imaging Study. J Neurotrauma 2021;38(16):2255–63.

107. Castaño Leon AM, Cicuendez M, Navarro B, et al. What Can Be Learned from Diffusion Tensor Imaging from a Large Traumatic Brain Injury Cohort?: White Matter Integrity and Its Relationship with Outcome. J Neurotrauma 2018;35(20):2365–76.

108. Prohl AK, Scherrer B, Tomas-Fernandez X, et al. Reproducibility of Structural and Diffusion Tensor Imaging in the TACERN Multi-Center Study. Front Integr Neurosci 2019;13:24.

109. Shenton ME, Hamoda HM, Schneiderman JS, et al. A review of magnetic resonance imaging and diffusion tensor imaging findings in mild traumatic brain injury. Brain Imaging Behav 2012;6(2):137–92.

110. Niogi SN, Mukherjee P. Diffusion tensor imaging of mild traumatic brain injury. J Head Trauma Rehabil 2010;25(4):241–55.

111. Ware JB, Hart T, Whyte J, et al. Inter-subject variability of axonal injury in diffuse traumatic brain injury. J Neurotrauma 2017;34(14):2243–53.

112. Sbardella E, Tona F, Petsas N, et al. DTI measurements in multiple sclerosis: evaluation of brain damage and clinical implications. Multiple sclerosis international 2013;2013:671730.

113. Saatman KE, Duhaime AC, Bullock R, et al. Classification of traumatic brain injury for targeted therapies. J Neurotrauma 2008;25(7):719–38.

114. Jain KK. Neuroprotection in traumatic brain injury. Drug Discov Today 2008;13(23–24):1082–9.

115. Bullock MR, Lyeth BG, Muizelaar JP. Current status of neuroprotection trials for traumatic brain injury: lessons from animal models and clinical studies. Neurosurgery 1999;45(2):207–17. ; discussion 217-20.

116. Narayan RK, Michel ME, Ansell B, et al. Clinical trials in head injury. *Journal of neurotrauma*. May 2002;19(5):503–57.

117. Tolias CM, Bullock MR. Critical appraisal of neuroprotection trials in head injury: what have we learned? NeuroRx 2004;1(1):71–9.

118. Loane DJ, Faden AI. Neuroprotection for traumatic brain injury: translational challenges and emerging therapeutic strategies. Trends Pharmacol Sci 2010; 31(12):596–604.

119. Kaloostian P, Robertson C, Gopinath SP, et al. Outcome prediction within twelve hours after severe traumatic brain injury by quantitative cerebral blood flow. J Neurotrauma 2012;29(5):727–34.

120. Steven AJ, Zhuo J, Melhem ER. Diffusion kurtosis imaging: an emerging technique for evaluating the microstructural environment of the brain. AJR Am J Roentgenol 2014;202(1):W26–33.

121. Glenn GR, Kuo LW, Chao YP, et al. Mapping the Orientation of White Matter Fiber Bundles: A Comparative Study of Diffusion Tensor Imaging, Diffusional Kurtosis Imaging, and Diffusion

Spectrum Imaging. AJNR Am J Neuroradiol 2016; 37(7):1216–22.

122. Palacios EM, Owen JP, Yuh EL, et al. The evolution of white matter microstructural changes after mild traumatic brain injury: A longitudinal DTI and NODDI study. Sci Adv 2020;6(32):eaaz6892.

123. Grossman EJ, Ge Y, Jensen JH, et al. Thalamus and cognitive impairment in mild traumatic brain injury: a diffusional kurtosis imaging study. J Neurotrauma 2012;29(13):2318–27.

124. Asken BM, DeKosky ST, Clugston JR, et al. Diffusion tensor imaging (DTI) findings in adult civilian, military, and sport-related mild traumatic brain injury (mTBI): a systematic critical review. Brain Imaging Behav 2018;12(2):585–612.

125. Fagerholm ED, Hellyer PJ, Scott G, et al. Disconnection of network hubs and cognitive impairment after traumatic brain injury. Brain 2015;138(Pt 6): 1696–709.

126. Liu Y, Wang T, Chen X, et al. Tract-based Bayesian multivariate analysis of mild traumatic brain injury. Comput Math Methods Med 2014;2014:120182.

127. Grass V. Machine learning classification of traumatic brain injury patients versus healthy controls using arterial spin labeled perfusion MRI. New York: CUNY Academic Works; 2021.

128. Maleki N, Finkel A, Cai G, et al. Post-traumatic Headache and Mild Traumatic Brain Injury: Brain Networks and Connectivity. Curr Pain Headache Rep 2021;25(3):20.

129. Sharma A, Garner R, La Rocca M, et al. Machine Learning of Diffusion Weighted Imaging for Prediction of Seizure Susceptibility Following Traumatic Brain Injury 2021. Annual Modeling and Simulation Conference (ANNSIM), Fairfax, VA, USA, 2021, pp. 1–9, https://doi.org/10.23919/ANNSIM52504.2021.9552121.

130. Abdelrahman H, Shiho U, Ueda K, et al. Automated classification of traumatic brain injury using machine learning with multiple indices of Diffusion Tensor Imaging. IDRO Reports 2019,0.0100.

The Current State of Functional MR Imaging for Trauma Prognostication

Daniel Ryan, MD[a], Saeedeh Mirbagheri, MD[b],
Noushin Yahyavi-Firouz-Abadi, MD[c],*

KEYWORDS

- Functional MRI • Traumatic brain injury • Post-traumatic stress disorder • Coma
- Post-concussive syndrome

KEY POINTS

- Network activity changes from baseline are greatest in the first few weeks following a head injury and reflect an attempt the brain makes to compensate for the sentinel injury and the ensuing metabolic shift associated with healing
- The degree of alteration of brain activation or network connectivity change over time correlates with the severity of postconcussive symptoms and time to normalization and may be used for prognostication or treatment planning
- Heterogeneity in study design and limitations in sample sizes contribute to an imperfect representation of healing brain networks; however, rapid progress in accumulating data inspires optimism for a future of brain diagnostic, prognostic, and therapeutic capabilities

INTRODUCTION

Traumatic brain injury (TBI) has the largest influence on morbidity and mortality in trauma patients.[1] Mild-to-moderate concussive injuries affect more than 69 million people worldwide annually, and traumatic coma occurs in approximately 1 million people worldwide each year.[2] Mild-to-moderate TBI is the most common cause of neurologic injury among athletes and military personnel.[3] In total, the US health care expenses related to these traumatic deficits are estimated at $17 billion annually.[4] The health care costs of these injuries relate to cognitive impairment in the acute post-concussive state, which typically lasts up to 10 days after the injury and less commonly may continue for weeks to months as post-concussive syndrome (PCS).[5] Common concussion symptoms include headache, nausea, visual disturbance, imbalance, distractibility, delay in verbal expression/bradyphrenia,

memory disturbance/fogginess, sleep disturbance, and emotional lability.[6] Health care providers often advocate avoiding continued exposure to reinjury in the days to weeks following the initial insult, as patients that experience second impacts may go on to worse morbidity and mortality.[6] Primary injury to the brain is the result of direct impact and is followed by an inflammatory response with neurotransmitter release and vascular dysfunction.[7] Animal models demonstrate that neuronal energy metabolism disruption from aerobic to anaerobic partially triggered by overrelease of glutamate drives clinical symptoms in the days to weeks following the insult and may persist for up to 4 weeks post-injury (Fig. 1).[7] Hemodynamic and metabolic network activity shifts are of interest to investigators that use functional data and imaging to better understand the brain in its post-traumatic state.[1] These observations improve the understanding of brain network activity that conventional imaging lacks.

[a] Southern Illinois University School of Medicine, 401 East Carpenter Street, Springfield, IL, USA; [b] University of Vermont Medical Center, 111 Colchester Avenue, Burlington, VT 05401, USA; [c] University of Maryland School of Medicine, 22 South Greene Street, Baltimore, MD 21201, USA
* Corresponding author.
E-mail address: nyahyavi@gmail.com

Neuroimag Clin N Am 33 (2023) 299–313
https://doi.org/10.1016/j.nic.2023.01.005
1052-5149/23/Published by Elsevier Inc.

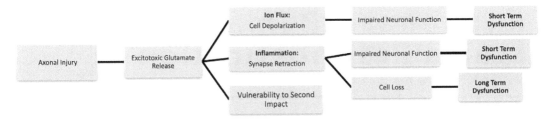

Fig. 1. Neurometabolic basis of traumatic brain injury.[8] (*Adapted from* Giza C, Greco T, Prins ML. Concussion: pathophysiology and clinical translation. Handb Clin Neurol. 2018;158:51-61.)

Limitations of Structural Imaging

Structural imaging modalities, such as computed tomography (CT) scans as well as MR imaging, are helpful in diagnosis and to some extent acute prognostication.[9] CT's sensitivity for detecting fractures and hemorrhages may provide large-scale structural information characteristic of moderate to severe TBI.[10] For parenchymal shear injuries that may be associated with microhemorrhage or tract swelling, 20% are recognized by CT and 80% by MR imaging.[11] A milder variety of partial shear injuries can be difficult to detect without significant hemorrhage or swelling but may longitudinally manifest through volume loss.[2] In addition, structural imaging techniques only characterize parenchymal abnormalities rather than provide a physiologic assessment of network activity that may better predict ongoing physical, cognitive, or emotional disability.[10] Therefore, functional imaging techniques have been beneficial in recognizing neural network disruption.[8] Furthermore, physiologic data could then be helpful in prognostication and evaluation of the effects of future therapies on brain networks. As a result, investigators are evaluating functional networks through electroencephalography (EEG), magnetic encephalography (MEG), and functional MRI (fMRI) to increase the sensitivity in recognizing injuries to brain networks that can influence clinical outcomes.[12] This review expands on the utility of fMRI to evaluate network activity, as well as patterns of injury and their clinical prognostic data.

BACKGROUND OF FUNCTIONAL MR IMAGING

Characterization and understanding of brain network activity have advanced tremendously as a result of Dr Bharat Biswal's recognition that low-frequency blood-oxygen-level-dependent (BOLD) signal fluctuations can be detected using sequential echo-planar MR imaging in 1995.[13] His team's research noticed focal BOLD signal intensity decrease corresponding to local increases in blood flow that increased the concentration of diamagnetic oxyhemoglobin compared with the baseline oxygen tension that is relatively paramagnetic.[14] Through BOLD imaging, the neurovascular coupling of network activity with increased local blood flow helps investigators demonstrate the energy demands necessary to sustain network function as well as piece together network components and characteristics.[13]

A typical hemodynamic response after neuronal activity that can accomplish neurovascular coupling involves a change in vascular tone within 500 ms and a peak in cerebrovascular dilatation approximately 3 to 5 s following the onset of activity.[15] These functions become more complex with increased duration and/or sequential activity where peak and plateau patterns may occur, and the hemodynamic response functions rely on local and remote vascular architecture, as well as potential pathomechanisms of cerebrovascular uncoupling.[16] As a result, the technique used in fMRI sequences captures images every 250 ms to observe these shifts related to neuronal activation.[17]

Certain design factors help organize network behavior around a relative state of rest (resting-state or rs-fMRI) or through periods of instructed activity such that investigators can observe network activity through segmental blocks, continuous event-related triggering, and continuous rapid event-related and mixed recording of data.[17] These iterations of study design uncover specific characteristics, such as similar frequencies in discrete brain regions at the same time, which suggests functional connectivity that over time may be seen as dynamic connectivity, or in a specific sequence of regional activation such as with effective connectivity of the brain's networks in their varied states of rest and activation.[18] Using different analysis methods, investigators can observe functionally connected brain regions, such as individual sensorimotor (or somatomotor), executive control, three visual, two lateral frontoparietal, auditory, and temporoparietal networks (Fig. 2, Table 1).[20]

Through appropriate design, studies can focus on differences between varied cognitive states

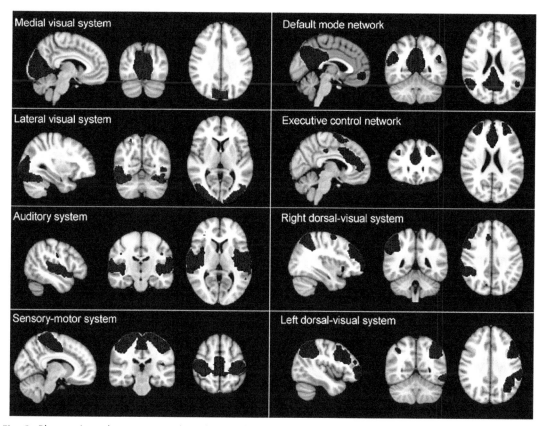

Fig. 2. Blue regions demonstrate selected spatially distinct areas of the brain that demonstrate synchronous BOLD fluctuations at rest (resting state functional networks). Original Figure previously published by Adriaanse and colleagues[19] in PLOS ONE. (*From* Adriaanse SM, Binnewijzend MA, Ossenkoppele R, et al. Widespread disruption of functional brain organization in early-onset Alzheimer's disease. PLoS One. 2014;9(7):e102995. Published 2014 Jul 31.)

(ie, subtraction), variations in similar cognitive processes (ie, factorial), variance in intensity of cognitive state (ie, parametric), and/or coexistence of variant cognitive processes (ie, conjunctional).[21] Interestingly, when investigators analyze network activity after subjects are instructed to perform tasks, task-specific networks are recruited and resting-state networks that integrate emotional and sensory information demonstrate suppression.[18] These observations not only teach us about adaptive prioritization of network activity but help reinforce the reactive and recompose cycles that underlie the brain's processing, and exemplify disordered resting-state or task-related network activity.[18]

In patients where task-based design is not a limitation, network activity comparison is best observed after periods of intention, recorded as blocks, events, or mixed-block events recording the subject performing tasks for an interval separated by a period of rest.[22] Because task-based fMRI (tb-fMRI) requires appropriate auditory processing, language fluency, comprehension, alertness, and

ability to carry out instructions, resting-state examinations may be more suitable for people with language barriers, those who have the inability to perceive or process instructions, those with difficulty with maintaining attention to instructions, those with mental illness, those in a vegetative state, or those with the physical inability to accomplish tasks, among other reasons.[23] The block design also enables a variety of pre-processing methods to correct for potential section-dependent time shifts, intensity differences, head motion, and/or cardiac/respiratory noise.[24] Whole-brain regression models may average time course or seed regions of interest to areas of activity in other regions by establishing boundary thresholds.[25] Identifying components of networks provides further component analyses that can help decompose data into variables to find patterns of activity for network identification.[26] Transformations and clustering algorithms can plot and organize data into hierarchical, K-means, c-means, and graph-based displays to evaluate, compare, and demonstrate features of dependence of networks within or between individuals.[26] As a

Table 1
Common resting state network functions and involved regions of the brain

Network	Regions of Connectivity	Function
Default Mode Network (DMN)	• Ventromedial prefrontal cortex • Inferior parietal lobe • Posterior cingulate cortex • Precuneus	Self-referential/mind-wandering aspects of cognition
Central Executive Network	• Dorsolateral prefrontal cortex • Bilateral inferior, middle, and superior frontal cortices • Inferior parietal lobule • Anterior cingulate cortex (ACC)/supplementary motor area (SMA) • Bilateral insular cortices	High-level cognitive/executive function
Salience Network	• Dorsal anterior cingulate cortex • Anterior insula (fronto-insular) connections to subcortical and limbic structures	Attention to biological stimuli
Auditory Network	• Primary and secondary auditory cortices, including Heschl's gyrus • Bilateral superior temporal gyri • Posterior insular cortex	Audition (tone/pitch distinction), music, speech
Sensorimotor Network	• Supplementary motor area/midcingulate cortex • Bilateral primary motor cortex • Bilateral middle frontal gyri	Motor tasks

result, scrutiny in methods of data acquisition and processing is of utmost importance as each method is associated with data transformation or has assumptions applied to the data that alter our analysis of network activity.[27]

FINDINGS IN FUNCTIONAL MR IMAGING

Tb-fMRI has been helpful in diagnosing, characterizing, and predicting the severity of deficits in specific functions such as learning/memory, motor, and cognition in trauma patients. Rs-fMRI is often easier to perform than tb-fMRI in trauma patients with alterations in mental status or children and provides information on changes in the network connectivity of the brain. fMRI has been used to assess the chronologic changes in brain function in trauma and has a potential for prognostication of recovery. We searched PubMed for all the studies using fMRI techniques in trauma patients (a total of 1253 articles) and found 504 articles relevant to rs-fMRI and tb-fMRI in the setting of trauma. Here, we have summarized the studies with a longitudinal design (at least two fMRI studies in different time standpoints) in Table 2 (rs-fMRI) and Table 3 (tb-fMRI). These studies have variations in results

that can be attributed to factors including age, individual variability, gender, the severity of the trauma, and more importantly study design (timing of scans, scan parameters, and analysis techniques). However, some general trends have been identified.

Default Mode Network: Some investigators have found increased connectivity and cerebral blood flow during the first 3 to 5 days after injury within portions of the default mode network, such as the hippocampus, which later may show reduced connectivity.[60] Patients with chronic PCS over multiple stages of recovery have demonstrated an overall imbalance in the ratio of cerebral blood flow between the default mode network and the task-positive networks suggesting that alterations in perfusion may underlie and predict chronic morbidity.[33] A traumatically decreased synchronization of neurons often requires an overall increased need for global connectivity to maintain signals as well as an increased metabolic need with increased cerebral blood flow and without this increase in blood flow prolonged impairment may occur.[32,34]

As a result, decreased fractional amplitude of low-frequency fluctuations within the motor, default-mode, and visual networks measured less than 10 days after injury with resting-state fMRI were

Table 2
Summary of longitudinal resting-state functional MR imaging studies in trauma patients

Study's First Author and Year	Participants	Timing of Scan	Findings
Harnett et al,[28] 2021	109 mTBI patients average age 35.31 y	~2 wk and 3 mo	• Left dorsolateral prefrontal cortex to arousal network connectivity at 2 wk post-trauma was negatively related to 3-mo PTSD symptoms and depression. • Right inferior temporal gyrus to DMN connectivity was positively related to 3-mo PTSD symptoms and depression. • Following trauma exposure, acutely assessed variability in RSN connectivity was associated with PTSD symptom severity approximately two and a half months later. • Decreased top-down cortico-limbic regulation and increased network-mediated fear generalization might contribute to dysfunction in the aftermath of trauma.
Manning et al,[29] 2017	31 concussed Hockey players aged 11 to 14 y	24 to 72 h ($n = 17$) and 3 mo ($n = 14$)	• Increased connectivity at 3 mo in sensorimotor, cerebellar, and DMN compared with 24 to 72 h • The adolescent brain may be more vulnerable to brain dysfunction and elongated periods of recovery after an acceleration-related injury.
Chong et al,[30] 2019	15 patients aged 16 to 55 with mTBI	1 and 5 mo	• At 1 mo post-concussion, patients had significantly weaker homotopic functional connectivity in several pain-processing regions which showed significant recovery at 5 mo. Better symptom recovery is associated with better functional somatosensory improvement.
Moreira da Silva et al,[31] 2020	23 mild-to-moderate TBI, median age of 36	6 d, 12 mo	• Sixteen brain network metrics were found to be discriminative of different post-injury phases. Eleven of those explain 90% of the variability observed in cognitive recovery following TBI.

(continued on next page)

Table 2
(continued)

Study's First Author and Year	Participants	Timing of Scan	Findings
			• Brain network metrics that had a high contribution to the explained variance were found in the frontal and temporal cortex, as well as the anterior cingulate cortex. This suggests that network reorganization may be related to the recovery of impaired cognitive function in the first year after a TBI.
Meier et al,[32] 2017	43 collegiate athletes concussion	1 d, 1 wk, 1 mo	• Regional homogeneity (ReHo) in sensorimotor, visual, and temporal cortices increased over time post-concussion and was greatest at 1-month post-injury. • ReHo in the frontal cortex decreased over time following concussion, with the greatest decrease evident at 1-month post-concussion. • Results are suggestive of delayed onset of local connectivity changes with no change in global connectivity following concussion
Sours et al,[33] 2015	28 patients, 28 controls average age 39 mTBI	11 d, 1 mo, ~6 mo	• Chronic mTBI patients with normalized cognitive performance, demonstrate increased resting-state connectivity (rs-FC) between the DMN and regions associated with the salience network and task-positive networks, as well as reduced strength of rs-FC within the DMN at the acute stage of injury. • Patients with chronic PCS reveal an imbalance in the ratio of cerebral blood flow between the DMN nodes and task-positive nodes across multiple stages of recovery. • Altered network perfusion with the associated changes in connectivity may be a possible predictor of which mTBI patients will develop chronic PCS.

(continued on next page)

Table 2
(continued)

Study's First Author and Year	Participants	Timing of Scan	Findings
Churchill et al,[34] 2020	228 university athletes, 61 concussion, 167 control average age 20	Acute (1 to 7 d), subacute (8 to 14 d), clearance to return to sport (RTS), 1 mo post-RTS and 1 y post-RTS	• BOLD scale-free signal (c1) was lowest at the acute injury, became significantly increased at RTS, and returned near control levels by 1-y post-RTS. • Clinical measures of acute symptom severity and time to RTP were related to longitudinal changes in c(1). Athletes with both greater symptoms and prolonged recovery had elevated c(1) values at RTS, while athletes with greater symptoms but rapid recovery had reduced c(1) at the acute injury.
Churchill et al,[35] 2021	167 university athletes age 20 monitored for 5 y	Baseline, concussed in the same season, ($n = 17$), concussed in later seasons ($n = 15$)	• Prior to the injury, concussed in the same season athletes had significantly elevated total symptom severity scores and elevated salience-DMN network rs-FC. • Salience-DMN network connectivity are associated with short-term but not long-term concussion risk.
Madhavan et al,[36] 2019	91 mTBI 15 to 51 y	<3 d, 5 to 10 d, 15 to 30 d and, 83 to 103 d	• Decreased fractional amplitude of low-frequency fluctuations (fALFF) was observed in specific functional networks for patients with higher symptom severity scores and fALFF returned to higher values when the patient recovered. • Functional connectivity immediately after injury was capable of predicting symptom severity at a later time. • Connectivity between motor, default-mode, and visual predicted 3-mo clinical outcome.
Dall'Acqua et al,[37] 2017	49 mTBI and 49 healthy controls mean age 35	5 d and 1 y	• Early phase: functional hypoconnectivity in default mode network. • One year: partial normalization which correlated with improvements in working memory, divided attention, and verbal recall.

(continued on next page)

Table 2
(*continued*)

Study's First Author and Year	Participants	Timing of Scan	Findings
Abbas et al,[38] 2015	10 male high school football athletes	Baseline, two in-season within 48 h of the game (2 months), six post-season	• In-season DMN connections were reduced in the first month and increased in the second month. • Post-Season connections were significantly reduced at all sessions except the December measurements.
Sours et al,[39] 2015	32 mTBI patients (15 with PCS	10 d, 6 mo	• Decreased strength of DMN connectivity within 0.125 to 0.250 Hz frequency range in patients with PCS compared with patients without the syndrome during both the acute and chronic phases.
Stephens et al,[40] 2018	17 children (10 to 17 y), mild–moderate TBI	2 mo, 12 mo	• Decreased anti-correlated functional connectivity between DMN and right Brodmann Area 40. • Worse performance on response inhibition tasks linked to more anomalous less anti-correlated connectivity between DMN and right Brodmann Area 40.
Johnson et al,[41] 2014	24 current collegiate rugby players	Baseline, 24 h after play	• DMN: increased connectivity from the left supramarginal gyrus to the bilateral orbitofrontal cortex and decreased connectivity from the retrosplenial cortex and dorsal posterior cingulate cortex. • Decreased functional connectivity after subconcussive head trauma in those with a history of trauma, while increased connectivity in those with no history.
Zhu et al,[42] 2015	8 concussed football athletes and 11 controls	within 24 h, 7 ± 1 d, and 30 ± 1 d after concussion	• Increased DMN functional connectivity on Day 1, a significant drop on Day 7, and partial recovery on Day 30
Kuceyeski et al,[43] 2019	26 mTBI (29.4 ± 8.0 y)	1 mo, 6-mo	• Increased functional connectome integration was related to better cognition recovery
Roy et al,[44] 2017	14 patients with moderate and severe TBI age 18 to 36	3, 6, and 12 mo following injury	• Increased network strength early after injury, but by 1-year post injury, hyperconnectivity was more circumscribed to frontal DMN and temporal-parietal attentional control regions.

(*continued on next page*)

Table 2
(continued)

Study's First Author and Year	Participants	Timing of Scan	Findings
Threlkeld et al,[45] 2018	17 acute severe TBI ICU patients, 16 healthy control	Acute imaging in all, 8 returned in 6 mo	• Acute: Those who remained in coma showed no DMN inter-network correlations. Those who recovered from coma to a minimally conscious or confusional state illustrated partially preserved DMN correlations. • Patients who recovered beyond the confusional state by 6 mo showed normal DMN correlations and anticorrelations similar to healthy subjects. • Recovery of consciousness after acute severe TBI is associated with partial preservation of DMN correlations in the ICU, followed by long-term normalization of DMN correlations and anticorrelations.
Hillary et al,[46] 2014	21 moderate and severe TBI and 15 controls	3 and 6 mo	• Hyperconnectivity during the first year disproportionately represented in the brain's core subnetworks.
vanderHorn et al,[47] 2017	30 mTBI patients and 20 control	1 mo and 3 mo post-injury	• Increased functional connectivity between the anterior and posterior components of the DMN at 1 mo post-injury was associated with a larger number of complaints at 3 mo post-injury.
Nakamura et al,[48] 2009	6 patients with severe TBI	3 mo and 6 mo	• Decreased strength of network connectivity from 3 mo to 6 mo post-injury.

associated with increased symptom severity and were useful in predicting 3 weeks to 3 months symptom severity.[36] Functional hypo-connectivity among regions involving the default mode network and hyper-connectivity in regions including cingulate cortex during the early phase of mTBI correlated well with early symptom severity.[37] However, 2-week post-injury connectivity of the left dorsolateral prefrontal cortex and the arousal network (amygdala, hippocampus, mammillary bodies, midbrain, and pons) was negatively associated with 3-month PTSD, in contrast to the connectivity of the right inferior temporal gyrus and default mode network which was positively correlated with 3-month PTSD and depression symptoms.[28]

Task Positive Networks: Interestingly, regional hyperactivation of task-positive networks, such as regions involved in working memory tasks, have been associated with persistent cognitive symptoms lasting beyond 1 week after injury.[53] In a group of adolescents with moderate to severe TBI exposed to varying difficulty working memory loads, lower response accuracy and longer reaction times were associated with elevated activity in the anterior cingulate gyrus and decreased activity in the left sensorimotor region that was relatively normalized on retesting 12 months later.[49] Even among patients with no reported deficit significantly higher activity within the parietal cortex, right dorsolateral prefrontal cortex, and right hippocampus

Table 3
Summary of longitudinal task-based functional MR imaging studies in trauma patients

Study's First Author and Year	Participants	Timing of Scans	Paradigm	Findings
Cazalis et al,[49] 2011	Adolescents (13 to 18 y of age) with moderate to severe TBI	Acute and 12 mo	Spatial working memory task	• Over 12 mo, patients' behavioral performance improved, suggesting cognitive recovery and patients recruited less of the anterior cingulate gyrus and more of the left sensorimotor cortex with increasing task difficulty.
Sanchez-Carrion et al,[50] 2008	12 patients with severe TBI, 10 control	Twice at a 6-mo interval	Working memory	• Low activation of the right superior frontal gyrus in the TBI group, with near resolution at 6 mo.
Chen et al,[51] 2012	20 mTBI and 18 healthy controls	Within 1 mo after injury and 6 wk later	Working memory	• Impaired increase in activation in working memory circuitry under both moderate and high working memory load conditions which improved at 6 mo. Able to detect abnormality in mTBI patient with normal neurobehavioral test.
Dettwiller et al,[52] 2014	15 athletes (mean age 20) 7 with concussion	3 d, 2 wk, and 2 mo post-injury after a concussion	Verbal/spatial working memory task	• Increased activation in bilateral dorsolateral prefrontal cortex in all time points and in inferior parietal lobe in 3 d and 2 weeks in the concussed group while normal standard working task.
Wylie et al,[53] 2015	27 Adult mTBI, 19 control	< 72 h, 1-wk	Working memory	• Increase in activation of posterior cingulate in mTBI subjects compared with controls which were greater in those without cognitive recovery.
Lovell et al,[54] 2007	28 concussed, 13 controls between (age 13 to 24)	Within 1 wk, after clinical recovery	Working memory	• Twice longer recovery time in athletes with a higher degree of activation of middle and inferior frontal cortex.

Study	Sample	Time points	Task	Findings
Hsu et al,[55] 2015	30 mTBI (15 M, 15 F), 30 control	Within 1 mo, 6 wk after the first study	Working memory	• Hyperactivation in male and hypoactivation in female patients initially which improved in male patients but persisted in female patients.
Coffey et al,[56] 2021	8 patients severe TBI	Acute, 6 mo	Speech	• Re-emergence of language-processing cortex activity by 6 mo in those with recovered language function.
Kim et al,[57] 2009	17 TBI, 15 control	Acute, repeat in 10 after cognitive rehabilitation	Visuospatial attention task	• Cognitive training in TBI patients improved performance of attention tasks and networks by increased activation of the anterior cingulate and precuneus.
Wu et al,[58] 2020	20 TB mild to severe	Acute and in 5 wk	Attention and working memory	• Increased activity patterns over time in the right dorsolateral prefrontal cortex and right insula. Decreased activity patterns in the left posterior cingulate cortex (PCC), bilateral precuneus, right inferior occipital gyrus, and right temporo-occipital junction.
Chen et al,[59] 2015	13 younger (mean 26 y), 13 older (mean 57 y) mTBI	1 mo, 6 wk later	Working memory	• Younger patients: initial hyperactivation in the right precuneus and right inferior parietal gyrus; Older patients: hypoactivation in the right precuneus and right inferior frontal gyrus. • Increased activation associated with increased postconcussion symptoms. • Partial recovery of activation pattern and decreased postconcussion symptoms in younger patients but not in older patients.

were demonstrated after visual and spatial memory tasks suggesting a reduced ability to recruit additional neuronal network power that may be indicative of early reorganization.[30,38] As a result, increased functional connectivity or reduced relative regional homogeneity in the right frontoparietal network were linked to elevated awareness of external stimuli and associated with increased cognitive fatigue even if it normalized 6 months later as working memory improved.[32,50]

These findings suggest that a temporal window of a few weeks to months is available for the brain to reorganize its connectivity by increasing the overall numbers of connections that have different frequency characteristics to account for the decreased strength of previously few but strong functional connections.[31] Despite this, some regions such as the hippocampus have a greater difficulty reorganizing and demonstrate reduced hippocampal volume and corresponding regional neural activity similar to that of patients of older age.[61] An individual's baseline introspective strength and adeptness at task performance may define how susceptible one is to dysfunction and the potential emotional sequelae of injury.[62] As a result, excess reactivity of threat-detection and fear-response regions of the brain after injury or exposure to psychological trauma, such as the amygdala, insula, and dorsal anterior cingulate cortex, as well as low-reward reactivity in affect-evaluation regions, such as the nucleus accumbens, amygdala, and orbitofrontal cortex, have been associated with higher stress vulnerability and elevated likelihood for chronic depression and post-traumatic stress disorders.[63]

Most tb-fMRI studies have assessed the working memory and to lesser extent attention and speech activation in the acute to the chronic setting (see Table 2). There is a general trend of cortical hyperactivation in the acute setting that improves over time. TBI patients have increased activation of the posterior cingulate gyrus[49,53] dorsolateral prefrontal cortex,[52] and inferior parietal lobe[59] with memory tasks, which improves over time. Interestingly, even in patients with mTBI and normal neurocognitive testing, there may be abnormal activation of task-related networks.[51] The degree of hyperactivation is a negative prognostic factor for normalization and the length of time needed for the recovery of cognitive abilities[53,54] and is associated with worse postconcussive symptoms.[59]

SUMMARY AND FUTURE DIRECTIONS

Multiple studies have demonstrated that in the first few weeks following an injury, the brain makes its greatest shift in network activity that likely reflects a microstructural reorganization in an attempt to compensate for damaged connections. Longitudinal fMRI studies demonstrate a correlation between the degree of hyperactivation and network shifts in connectivity and post-concussive symptoms that may be helpful for predicting time to recovery, such as determining the timing to return to sport. In the future, genetic and injury-related fMRI clinical markers might stratify an individual's risk of ensuing morbidity that may guide neurochemical or ion channel-modulating therapeutic options or potential stem cell therapies. Current heterogeneity between study designs as well as limitations in sample sizes contributes to an imperfect representation of the healing brain networks. By normalizing fMRI as a regular evaluation for extended follow-up on trauma patients as well as refining inclusion criteria to decrease heterogeneity in the investigation of TBI, investigators could achieve an unprecedented advancement of neural health and science that may extend beyond the setting of trauma.

CLINICS CARE POINTS

- In the first few weeks following an injury, the brain makes its greatest shift in network activity that likely reflects a microstructural reorganization in an attempt to compensate for damaged connections.
- Some brain regions are less versatile than others.
- Longitudinal fMRI studies demonstrate a correlation between the degree of hyperactivation and network shifts in connectivity and post-concussive symptoms that may be helpful for predicting time to recovery, such as determining the timing to return to sport.
- Current heterogeneity between study designs as well as limitations in sample sizes contributes to an imperfect representation of the healing brain networks.

DISCLOSURE

None of the authors have any commercial or financial conflict of interest related to this article.

REFERENCES

1. Cristofori I, Levin HS. Traumatic brain injury and cognition. In: Grafman J, Salazar AM, editors. Handbook of

clinical neurology. Waltham, MA: Elsevier; Vol. 128, 2015. p. 579–611.

2. Edlow BL, Giacino JT, Wu O. Functional MRI and Outcome in Traumatic Coma. Curr Neurol Neurosci Rep 2013;13(9):375.

3. Dewan MC, Rattani A, Gupta S, et al. Estimating the global incidence of traumatic brain injury. J Neurosurg 2019;130(4):1080–97.

4. Archer KR, Coronado RA, Haislip LR, et al. Telephone-based goal management training for adults with mild traumatic brain injury: Study protocol for a randomized controlled trial. Trials 2015;16(1):244.

5. Maroon JC, LePere DB, Blaylock RL, et al. Postconcussion Syndrome: A Review of Pathophysiology and Potential Nonpharmacological Approaches to Treatment. Physician and Sportsmedicine 2012;40(4):73–87.

6. McCrory P, Meeuwisse W, Dvorak J, et al. Consensus statement on concussion in sport—The 5 th international conference on concussion in sport held in Berlin, October 2016. Br J Sports Med 2017; 51(11):838–47.

7. Halstead ME, Walter KD, Moffatt K. Sport-Related Concussion in Children and Adolescents. Pediatrics 2018;142(6):e20183074.

8. Giza C, Greco T, Prins ML. Concussion: pathophysiology and clinical translation. In: Hainline B, Stern RA, editors. Handbook of clinical neurology. Cambridge, MA: Elsevier; Vol. 158, 2018. p. 51–61.

9. Mishra R, Ucros HEV, Florez-Perdomo WA, et al. Predictive Value of Rotterdam Score and Marshall Score in Traumatic Brain Injury: A Contemporary Review. Indian J Neurotrauma 2021;0041:1727404.

10. Raj R, Skrifvars M, Bendel S, et al. Predicting six-month mortality of patients with traumatic brain injury: Usefulness of common intensive care severity scores. Crit Care 2014;18(2):R60.

11. Palacios EM, Owen JP, Yuh EL, et al. The evolution of white matter microstructural changes after mild traumatic brain injury: A longitudinal DTI and NODDI study. Sci Adv 2020;6(32):eaaz6892.

12. Ianof JN, Anghinah R. Traumatic brain injury: An EEG point of view. Demen Neuropsychologia 2017; 11(1):3–5.

13. Hillman EMC. Coupling Mechanism and Significance of the BOLD Signal: A Status Report. Annu Rev Neurosci 2014;37(1):161–81.

14. Raichle ME. Behind the scenes of functional brain imaging: A historical and physiological perspective. Proc Natl Acad Sci 1998;95(3):765–72.

15. Hirano Y, Stefanovic B, Silva AC. Spatiotemporal Evolution of the Functional Magnetic Resonance Imaging Response to Ultrashort Stimuli. J Neurosci 2011;31(4):1440–7.

16. Biswal B, Zerrin Yetkin F, Haughton VM, et al. Functional connectivity in the motor cortex of resting human brain using echo-planar mri. Magn Reson Med 1995;34(4):537–41.

17. Zhang S, Li X, Lv J, et al. Characterizing and differentiating task-based and resting state fMRI signals via two-stage sparse representations. Brain Imaging Behav 2016;10(1):21–32.

18. Fox MD, Grecius M. Clinical applications of resting state functional connectivity. Front Syst Neurosci 2010;4(19):1–13.

19. Adriaanse SM, Binnewijzend MAA, Ossenkoppele R, et al. Widespread Disruption of Functional Brain Organization in Early-Onset Alzheimer's Disease. PLoS ONE 2014;9(7):e102995.

20. Mohan A, Roberto AJ, Mohan A, et al. The Significance of the Default Mode Network (DMN) in Neurological and Neuropsychiatric Disorders: A Review. Yale J Biol Med 2016;89(1):49–57.

21. Glover GH. Overview of Functional Magnetic Resonance Imaging. Neurosurg Clin N Am 2011;22(2): 133–9.

22. Esteban O, Ciric R, Finc K, et al. Analysis of task-based functional MRI data preprocessed with fMRIPrep. Nat Protoc 2020;15(7):2186–202.

23. Bennett CM, Miller MB. fMRI reliability: Influences of task and experimental design. Cogn Affective, Behav Neurosci 2013;13(4):690–702.

24. Park HJ, Friston KJ, Pae C, et al. Dynamic effective connectivity in resting state fMRI. NeuroImage 2018; 180:594–608.

25. Calhoun VD, Adali T. Unmixing fMRI with independent component analysis. IEEE Eng Med Biol Mag 2006;25(2):79–90.

26. Lee MH, Smyser CD, Shimony JS. Resting-State fMRI: A Review of Methods and Clinical Applications. Am J Neuroradiology 2013;34(10):1866–72.

27. Edlow BL, Rosenthal ES. Diagnostic, Prognostic, and Advanced Imaging in Severe Traumatic Brain Injury. Curr Trauma Rep 2015;1(3):133–46.

28. Harnett NG, van Rooij SJH, Ely TD, et al. Prognostic neuroimaging biomarkers of trauma-related psychopathology: Resting-state fMRI shortly after trauma predicts future PTSD and depression symptoms in the AURORA study. Neuropsychopharmacology 2021;46(7):1263–71.

29. Manning KY, Schranz A, Bartha R, et al. Multiparametric MRI changes persist beyond recovery in concussed adolescent hockey players. Neurology 2017;89(21):2157–66.

30. Chong CD, Wang L, Wang K, et al. Homotopic region connectivity during concussion recovery: A longitudinal fMRI study. PLoS ONE 2019;14(10): e0221892.

31. Moreira da Silva N, Cowie CJA, Blamire AM, et al. Investigating Brain Network Changes and Their Association With Cognitive Recovery After Traumatic Brain Injury: A Longitudinal Analysis. Front Neurol 2020;11:369.

32. Meier TB, Bellgowan PS, Mayer AR. Longitudinal assessment of local and global functional connectivity

following sports-related concussion. Brain Imaging Behav 2017;11(1):129–40.

33. Sours C, Zhuo J, Roys S, et al. Disruptions in Resting State Functional Connectivity and Cerebral Blood Flow in Mild Traumatic Brain Injury Patients. PLoS ONE 2015;10(8):e0134019.

34. Churchill NW, Hutchison MG, Graham SJ, et al. Scale-free functional brain dynamics during recovery from sport-related concussion. Hum Brain Mapp 2020;41(10):2567–82.

35. Churchill NW, Hutchison MG, Graham SJ, et al. Concussion Risk and Resilience: Relationships with Pre-Injury Salience Network Connectivity. J Neurotrauma 2021; 38(22):3097–106.

36. Madhavan R, Joel SE, Mullick R, et al. Longitudinal Resting State Functional Connectivity Predicts Clinical Outcome in Mild Traumatic Brain Injury. J Neurotrauma 2019;36(5):650–60.

37. Dall'Acqua P, Johannes S, Mica L, et al. Functional and Structural Network Recovery after Mild Traumatic Brain Injury: A 1-Year Longitudinal Study. Front Hum Neurosci 2017;11:280.

38. Abbas K, Shenk TE, Poole VN, et al. Effects of Repetitive Sub-Concussive Brain Injury on the Functional Connectivity of Default Mode Network in High School Football Athletes. Developmental Neuropsychol 2015;40(1):51–6.

39. Sours C, Chen H, Roys S, et al. Investigation of Multiple Frequency Ranges Using Discrete Wavelet Decomposition of Resting-State Functional Connectivity in Mild Traumatic Brain Injury Patients. Brain Connectivity 2015;5(7):442–50.

40. Stephens JA, Salorio CF, Barber AD, et al. Preliminary findings of altered functional connectivity of the default mode network linked to functional outcomes one year after pediatric traumatic brain injury. Developmental Neurorehabil 2018;21(7):423–30.

41. Johnson B, Neuberger T, Gay M, et al. Effects of Subconcussive Head Trauma on the Default Mode Network of the Brain. J Neurotrauma 2014;31(23):1907–13.

42. Zhu DC, Covassin T, Nogle S, et al. A Potential Biomarker in Sports-Related Concussion: Brain Functional Connectivity Alteration of the Default-Mode Network Measured with Longitudinal Resting-State fMRI over Thirty Days. J Neurotrauma 2015; 32(5):327–41.

43. Kuceyeski AF, Jamison KW, Owen JP, et al. Longitudinal increases in structural connectome segregation and functional connectome integration are associated with better recovery after mild TBI. Hum Brain Mapp 2019;40(15):4441–56.

44. Roy A, Bernier RA, Wang J, et al. The evolution of cost-efficiency in neural networks during recovery from traumatic brain injury. PLoS ONE 2017;12(4): e0170541.

45. Threlkeld ZD, Bodien YG, Rosenthal ES, et al. Functional networks reemerge during recovery of consciousness after acute severe traumatic brain injury. Cortex 2018;106:299–308.

46. Hillary FG, Rajtmajer SM, Roman CA, et al. The Rich Get Richer: Brain Injury Elicits Hyperconnectivity in Core Subnetworks. PLoS ONE 2014;9(8): e104021.

47. van der Horn HJ, Scheenen ME, de Koning ME, et al. The Default Mode Network as a Biomarker of Persistent Complaints after Mild Traumatic Brain Injury: A Longitudinal Functional Magnetic Resonance Imaging Study. J Neurotrauma 2017;34(23):3262–9.

48. Nakamura T, Hillary FG, Biswal BB. Resting Network Plasticity Following Brain Injury. PLoS ONE 2009; 4(12):e8220.

49. Cazalis F, Babikian T, Giza C, et al. Pivotal role of anterior cingulate cortex in working memory after traumatic brain injury in youth. Front Neurol 2011; 1(158):1–9.

50. Sanchez-Carrion R, Fernandez-Espejo D, Junque C, et al. A longitudinal fMRI study of working memory in severe TBI patients with diffuse axonal injury. NeuroImage 2008;43:421–9.

51. Chen CJ, Wu CH, Liao YP, et al. Working Memory in Patients with Mild Traumatic Brain Injury: Functional MR Imaging Analysis. Radiology 2012;264(3):844–51.

52. Dettwiler A, Murugavel M, Putukian M, et al. Persistent Differences in Patterns of Brain Activation after Sports-Related Concussion: A Longitudinal Functional Magnetic Resonance Imaging Study. J Neurotrauma 2014;31(2):180–8.

53. Wylie GR, Freeman K, Thomas A, et al. Cognitive improvement after mild traumatic brain injury measured with functional neuroimaging during the acute period. PLoS One 2015;10(5):e0126110.

54. Lovell MR, Pardini JE, Welling J, et al. Functional brain abnormalities are related to clinical recovery and time to return-to-play in athletes. Neurosurgery 2007;61(2):352–60.

55. Hsu HL, Chen DYT, Tseng YC, et al. Sex Differences in Working Memory after Mild Traumatic Brain Injury: A Functional MR Imaging Study. Radiology 2015; 276(3):828–35.

56. Coffey BJ, Threlkeld ZD, Foulkes AS, et al. Reemergence of the language network during recovery from severe traumatic brain injury: A pilot functional MRI study. Brain Inj 2021;35(11–12):1552–62.

57. Kim YH, Yoo WK, Ko MH, et al. Plasticity of the Attentional Network After Brain Injury and Cognitive Rehabilitation. Neurorehabil Neural Repair 2009;23(5): 468–77.

58. Wu SCJ, Jenkins LM, Apple AC, et al. Longitudinal fMRI task reveals neural plasticity in default mode network with disrupted executive-default coupling and selective attention after traumatic brain injury. Brain Imaging Behav 2020;14:1638–50.

59. Chen DYT, Hsu HL, Ying-Sheng Kuo YS, et al. Effect of Age on Working Memory Performance and

Cerebral Activation after Mild Traumatic Brain Injury: A Functional MR Imaging Study. Radiology 2015; 278(3):854–62.

60. Churchill NW, Hutchison MG, Richards D, et al. The first week after concussion: Blood flow, brain function and white matter microstructure. NeuroImage 2017;14:480–9.

61. Monti JM, Voss MW, Pence A, et al. History of mild traumatic brain injury is associated with deficits in relational memory, reduced hippocampal volume, and less neural activity later in life. Front Aging Neurosci 2013;5(41):1–9.

62. Feis RA, Bouts MJRJ, Dopper EGP, et al. Multimodal MRI of grey matter, white matter, and functional connectivity in cognitively healthy mutation carriers at risk for frontotemporal dementia and Alzheimer's disease. BMC Neurol 2019;19(1):343.

63. Stevens JS, Harnett NG, Lebois LAM, et al. Brain-Based Biotypes of Psychiatric Vulnerability in the Acute Aftermath of Trauma. Am J Psychiatry 2021; 178(11):1037–49.

Perfusion Imaging of Traumatic Brain Injury

Nathan W. Churchill, PhD[a,c,e,*], Simon J. Graham, PhD[b,f,g], Tom A. Schweizer, PhD[a,c,d]

KEYWORDS

• TBI • Concussion • Perfusion • Cerebral blood flow • MRI • CT

KEY POINTS

- Cerebral blood flow (CBF) is vulnerable to the effects of traumatic brain injury (TBI).
- Perfusion imaging techniques measure post-TBI deficits in CBF.
- CBF issues may underlie clinical outcomes across the injury severity spectrum.
- Imaging techniques are promising but not yet widely used in clinical settings.

INTRODUCTION

Traumatic brain injury (TBI) is a leading cause of morbidity and mortality worldwide, contributing to ~30% of all injury-related deaths.[1] It is increasingly recognized that multiple, complex neurophysiological disruptions occur during TBI that contribute to clinical outcomes. Cerebral perfusion is particularly noteworthy, given its critical role in brain function. In the healthy brain, tightly coordinated regulatory mechanisms ensure adequate blood flow to brain tissues, in the presence of time-varying metabolism and blood gas concentrations while buffering out other physiological effects such as fluctuations in arterial blood pressure.[2] Consequently, the disruption of mechanisms regulating blood flow may have profoundly negative consequences for those who suffer a TBI, across the spectrum of severe, moderate, and mild injury,[3] with the latter definition often encompassing concussion. There is strong evidence supporting the use of perfusion imaging techniques to identify these deficits in order to better inform and guide patient management.

This article reviews the role of cerebral perfusion imaging in TBI. First, mechanisms regulating normal perfusion in the brain are discussed, followed by TBI-related changes in perfusion, including pathophysiologic mechanisms and their natural evolution after injury. Next, established perfusion imaging techniques are reviewed along with their advantages and drawbacks, and the relevance of perfusion imaging is examined in three key TBI domains: (1) moderate-to-severe TBI and acute management, (2) mild TBI and persistent symptoms, and (3) sport concussion and safe return to play. This article then concludes by summarizing the current role of perfusion imaging in TBI and future applications.

MECHANISMS OF NORMAL PERFUSION

Cerebral perfusion refers to the amount of blood delivered to neural tissue to meet metabolic demands and is typically measured as cerebral blood flow (CBF), which equals the blood volume delivered to a mass of tissue per unit time, usually in units of milliliters per 100 grams of tissue per minute (mL/100 g/min). In healthy adults, global CBF is ~50 mL/100 g/min, whereas values below ~20 mL/100 g/min cause neural dysfunction and values below

[a] Neuroscience Research Program, Saint Michael's Hospital, 209 Victoria Street, Toronto, ON M5B 1M8, Canada; [b] Department of Medical Biophysics, University of Toronto, 101 College Street, Suite 15-701, Toronto, ON M5G 1L7, Canada; [c] Keenan Research Centre for Biomedical Science of St. Michael's Hospital, 209 Victoria Street, Toronto, ON M5B 1M8, Canada; [d] Faculty of Medicine (Neurosurgery), University of Toronto, 1 King's College Circle, Toronto, ON M5S 1A8, Canada; [e] Physics Department, Toronto Metropolitan University, 60 St George St, Toronto, ON M5S 1A7, Canada; [f] Hurvitz Brain Sciences Program, Sunnybrook Research Institute, Wellness Way, Toronto, ON M4N 3M5, Canada; [g] Physical Sciences Platform, Sunnybrook Research Institute, 2075 Bayview Avenue, Toronto, ON M4N 3M5, Canada
* Corresponding author. Neuroscience Research Program, Saint Michael's Hospital, 209 Victoria Street, Toronto, ON M5B 1M8.
E-mail address: nathan.churchill@unityhealth.to

Neuroimag Clin N Am 33 (2023) 315–324
https://doi.org/10.1016/j.nic.2023.01.006

~ 10 mL/100 g/min cause cell death within minutes,[4] although the threshold for irreversible damage may vary between different pathologies.[5] Blood flow is driven by cerebral perfusion pressure (CPP), which is defined as the difference in intracranial pressure (ICP) relative to mean arterial pressure. Cerebral autoregulation ensures consistent CBF in the presence of time-varying metabolic demands and fluctuations in systemic blood pressure. This autoregulation is achieved by altering cerebrovascular resistance through changes in vessel diameter of cerebral arterioles and capillary beds.[6] For example, reduced systemic blood pressure prompts a vasodilatory response to reduce vascular resistance and avoid CBF deficit, whereas increased blood pressure produces vasoconstriction to limit excess CBF. These mechanisms maintain consistent CBF across a wide range of CPP values, typically 50 to 150 mm Hg in healthy adults.[7] Outside this range, vasodilatory/vasoconstrictive capabilities can no longer buffer the effects of further changes in the blood pressure, causing CBF to vary passively with CPP. Decreases in CBF below autoregulatory limits therefore put an individual at risk of ischemia, whereas highly elevated CBF results in elevated ICP with associated risk of injury to cerebral vessels.

EFFECTS OF TRAUMATIC BRAIN INJURY ON PERFUSION

It is well established that TBI has a disruptive effect on CBF and its regulatory mechanisms.[8,9] The literature on TBI and pathophysiology distinguishes between primary injury, caused by the traumatic event (eg, contusion, skull fracture, axonal injury), and secondary injury, whereby cascading physiological processes in response to the primary injury lead to further tissue damage (eg, metabolic dysregulation, neurotransmitter release, neuroinflammation), which often emerges hours to days later.[10] Although numerous reviews survey the different physiological mechanisms at play in TBI,[11,12] here the focus is on those contributing to CBF dysregulation and the resulting consequences.

Moderate-to-Severe Traumatic Brain Injury: Pathophysiologic Mechanisms

In moderate-to-severe TBI, the overarching clinical concern is maintenance of CPP,[13] which may be disrupted by multiple factors post-injury. Elevated ICP often contributes to reduced CPP and is exacerbated by many factors, including hypovolemia, arterial hypotension (eg, due to vascular trauma and/or disruption of neural cardiac control systems), microvascular injury, and edema.[2,14] The latter includes vasogenic contributions, due to permeation of the

endothelium and cytotoxic contributions, from the accumulation of intracellular water.[15] Hypoperfusion contributes to further blood–brain barrier breakdown via excitotoxic effects, neuroinflammation, and oxidative stresses[16] with ongoing detrimental effects on perfusion. The cerebral vasculature also shows a diminished ability to compensate for low CPP after injury with impaired autoregulation and vasoreactivity frequently observed.[2] These effects put the brain in a greater state of vulnerability to ischemic injury, with CBF falling below autoregulatory limits and subsequently causing impaired function, death of neural tissue, and elevated risk of mortality, with ischemia due to elevated ICP and edema comprising nearly half of all TBI-related deaths.[17] Among survivors, there are also long-lasting deficits in behavior and cognition, sometimes with ongoing or emerging deficits years after the primary injury.[18] Furthermore, elevated ICP not only contributes to ischemic injury but also produces pressure-related distortion and compression of tissues, with the brainstem particularly at risk, leading to respiratory failure and death if left untreated.[19] These effects establish the critical role of perfusion in post-TBI mortality and, among survivors, lasting functional deficits.

Moderate-to-Severe Traumatic Brain Injury: Natural Evolution

For patients assessed within the first 1 to 2 weeks post-injury, when they are still highly symptomatic, reduced CBF is commonly reported.[20–22] However, there is also substantial inter-individual variability in the affected brain regions[22] and the magnitude of CBF effects,[9,23] which can range from hypoperfusion to hyperperfusion. A longitudinal study examining TBI patients from 1 to 6 weeks post-injury reported that average CBF values were low relative to uninjured controls within the first week, with average decreases persisting at 6 weeks post-injury.[24] They also reported, however, that a subset of individuals showed recovery of CBF values at 2 to 3 weeks post-injury, along with improved neurological outcomes at 6-week follow-up. These studies highlight the variable, long-lasting nature of post-TBI perfusion deficits, although a restoration of normal values seems to correlate with improved clinical outcome (see Sections "Moderate-to-severe traumatic brain injury and acute management" and "Mild traumatic brain injury and persistent symptoms" for further details).

Mild Traumatic Brain Injury: Pathophysiologic Mechanisms

As the more severe mechanisms of injury are typically absent in mild TBI, the comparatively milder secondary effects (the "neurometabolic cascade") predominate, causing microvascular and axonal injury. As established mainly through preclinical research involving animal models, CBF is impaired after a mild TBI[25,26] and uncoupled with neurometabolism, failing to match the increased metabolic demand of restoring ionic homeostasis in injured neural cells.[27] This leads to an energy crisis, whereby the resulting oxidative stresses weaken the blood–brain barrier, with further negative effects on cerebrovascular function.[28,29] Other factors may variably contribute to altered CBF response after mild TBI, including the extent of primary microvascular injury.[30] Damage to the neurovascular unit also reduces autoregulatory capacity,[31] although the effects are often subtle in mild TBI and, in some cases, may be nonsignificant or even enhanced.[2] Disrupted autoregulation can cause CBF insufficiencies, subtle ischemia, and/or oxidative stresses. Collectively, these issues affect neural functioning, contributing to the transient behavioral disturbances that are typically seen after mild TBI.[32]

Mild Traumatic Brain Injury: Natural Evolution

As in moderate-to-severe TBI, perfusion imaging studies of mild TBI have shown variable effects within the first week of injury. This includes elevated CBF relative to controls,[33] reduced values,[34] and nonsignificant differences.[35] These findings again point toward a variable initial CBF response to injury, which evolves mainly over the first 1 to 2 weeks; a longitudinal study found within-subject declines from 1 to 8 days post-injury, and a cross-sectional study similarly found that individuals imaged 1 to 3 days post-injury had elevated CBF, whereas those imaged 5 to 7 days had reduced values. The findings agree with preclinical research reporting elevated CBF to match the demands of acute hypermetabolism, with a later dip due to metabolic impairments and neurovascular uncoupling.[36] For mild TBI, the related post-concussion symptoms typically resolve in this 1 to 2 week time interval,[37] although some individuals experience a more prolonged recovery.[38,39] Normalization of acute CBF disturbances seems over a similar timeline,[34,40] although some individuals show long-lasting disturbances[40] (see Section "Sport concussion and safe return to play" for further details) (Fig. 1).

PERFUSION IMAGING METHODS

Perfusion imaging methods measure the concentration of a tracer agent as it passes through the cerebrovasculature. Emphasis is placed on flow through microvessels (arterioles and capillaries), which is intimately associated with neurometabolism through the delivery of nutrients to tissues and removal of waste products. Different perfusion imaging methods use different tracers, which may consist of exogenous materials delivered via injection or inhalation (radioactive, radiopaque, or paramagnetic materials) or endogenous materials in blood (magnetically labeled water). Information about tracer delivery (eg, whether delivered as a bolus or steady-state infusion, baseline tracer concentration) and kinetics (eg, rates of diffusion out of vascular spaces, tracer signal decay) is then incorporated into kinetic models that relate the tracer signal to CBF and other complementary measures, including cerebral blood volume (CBV), bolus time-to-peak, and mean transit time (MTT). In this section, perfusion computed tomography (CT) and MR imaging methods are summarized in terms of their physical principles and trade-offs, with the latter divided into contrast-enhanced (exogenous tracer) and arterial spin labeling (ASL) (endogenous tracer) categories. Nonquantitative modalities, such as single photon emission computed tomography, and modalities requiring specialized infrastructure, such as Xenon (Xe)-CT and oxygen-15 PET, are reviewed elsewhere[41–43] and not included for brevity.

Perfusion Computed Tomography

CT uses rotating x-ray beams and detectors to image different projections of the head, which are combined computationally to create an overall image with signal contrast related to the x-ray attenuation properties of tissues. When a radiopaque tracer (typically an iodinated contrast agent[44]) is delivered via bolus injection, CT imaging is used to track the distribution of the agent and to quantify CBF. Perfusion CT is increasingly being recommended in clinical settings and is commonly adopted in the workup for disorders such as acute stroke.[45,46] Perfusion CT has the advantage of being highly accessible in most first-world hospital settings and does not require the use of radionuclides. However, the radiation dose associated with perfusion CT may be of concern depending on the severity of TBI and in cases of ongoing patient management for which repeated imaging may be required.

Contrast-Enhanced MR Imaging

When patients are placed in the bore of an MR imaging system, the hydrogen nuclei of tissue water molecules become magnetized by a large static magnetic field. Radiofrequency energy is subsequently used for spatially selective, resonant excitation of the magnetization, with additional spatial encoding provided by imaging gradients (spatially varying magnetic fields), after which the resulting

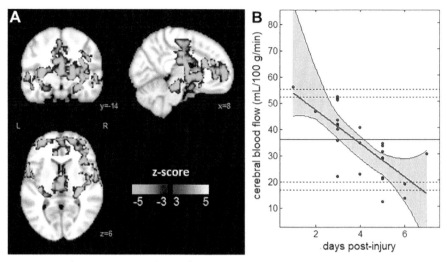

Fig. 1. Time varying early CBF response, shown for 26 participants with mild TBI. CBF is regressed against days post-injury, with (*A*) significant brain regions identified and (*B*) mean regional values plotted against days, with a group of 26 controls for comparison. In the latter panel, the line of best fit is plotted for the mild TBI group (solid red line) with 95% confidence bounds (pink shaded area); the mean control value is also plotted (solid black line) with 90% and 95% confidence bounds (dashed black lines). (*From* Churchill NW, Hutchison MG, Richards D, Leung G, Graham SJ, Schweizer TA. The first week after concussion: Blood flow, brain function and white matter microstructure. Neuroimage Clin. 2017;14:480-489. Published 2017 Feb 20.)

MR signals are converted into images. As with CT, contrast-enhanced MR imaging involves the injection of a tracer (typically gadolinium chelated to a macromolecule). Standard perfusion MR imaging is performed using the dynamic susceptibility contrast (DSC) method, in which passage of the gadolinium tracer through cerebrovasculature is measured as a transient decrease in T2*-weighted signal, which can then be used to estimate CBF and CBV.[47] Alternatively, the dynamic contrast-enhanced (DCE)-MR imaging method can also be used, in this case estimating CBF by the transient increase in T1-weighted signal.[48] Whereas DCE-MR imaging requires a lower tracer dose due to the increased sensitivity of the T1-weighted effect,[49] DSC-MR imaging has higher temporal resolution, which may be pertinent in cases of suspected intracranial hemorrhage. Although perfusion CT predominates in the clinical setting due to its relative affordability and accessibility, contrast-enhanced MR imaging offers equivalent information without ionizing radiation. In addition, contrast-enhanced MR imaging may be attractive due to the anatomical information provided in a typical MR imaging protocol, where signal contrast is usually superior to CT.

Arterial Spin Labeling

The ASL MR imaging method for estimating CBF is increasingly adopted in clinical applications. Rather than requiring an exogenous tracer, ASL uses radiofrequency excitation of water molecules flowing from arteries in the neck as the source of endogenous contrast. Thus, ASL is useful in cases where an exogenous contrast agent is contraindicated (eg, multiple organ trauma common to more severe TBI). The labeled water subsequently transits to capillary beds to produce a small but detectable change in regional MR imaging signal. The "labelled" image is then contrasted against an unlabeled "control" image.[50] The difference in signal intensity due to labeled water is proportional to CBF and can be converted to absolute units using a simple kinetic model.[51] Different labeling schemes exist, although the current consensus is that pseudo-continuous ASL[52] is preferred for clinical applications. Unfortunately, the ASL methods suffer from inherently low signal-to-noise ratio and sensitivity to motion due to the use of subtraction images, but major strides have been recently made to enhance robustness, making ASL a viable alternative to contrast-enhanced MR imaging.

MODERATE-TO-SEVERE TRAUMATIC BRAIN INJURY AND ACUTE MANAGEMENT

In hospital settings, patient management focuses on controlling secondary injury after TBI, which is mainly caused by hypoxia and arterial hypotension.[13] Rapid neurologic examinations are typically performed during intake, with severity stratification based on a calculated Glasgow Coma Scale (GCS) score. Those suspected of TBI then usually undergo non-contrast CT, depending on the presence of other injuries requiring more urgent attention. Subsequent monitoring of cerebrovascular function is oriented around the measurement of ICP and CPP intracranially, although these indices are inexact proxies of CBF.[53] Given the paramount importance of perfusion in patient recovery, usage of sophisticated perfusion imaging tools may be warranted in clinical management of TBI.

Large prospective studies, typically using perfusion CT, have identified significant associations between acute CBF and post-TBI outcomes. One such study found that the number of cerebral territories with reduced CBV was a significant predictor of 3-month outcome based on the Glasgow Outcome Scale (GOS).[54] Other studies using Xe-CT similarly found that both global and regional perfusion at acute injury were significantly predictive of postdischarge GOS scores,[55,56] although nonsignificant associations with GOS have also been reported.[23] Other studies have shown mixed results in terms of clinical utility, depending on the target outcome. Two studies failed to find associations between acute CBF and GCS at intake, reflecting the severity of initial trauma,[23,57] although higher CBF and lower MTT values were related to more favorable outcomes.[57] A recent feasibility study found that perfusion CT acquired within 48 hours of injury provided extremely high positive and negative predictive values for brain death[58]; whereas another study of comatose patients found acute CBF to be negatively correlated with risk of death/vegetative state, but only if cases of hyperperfusion were excluded from modeling.[9] There is also evidence for utility in the early identification of viable brain tissue, with acute perfusion CT showing significant correlations with non-contrast CT findings obtained 1 week later.[59] These studies provide substantial evidence supporting the role of perfusion imaging in managing moderate-to-severe TBI and predicting functional outcomes after injury.

MILD TRAUMATIC BRAIN INJURY AND PERSISTENT SYMPTOMS

On the milder end of the injury spectrum, individuals with mild TBI rarely present with significant neurological or radiological findings; hence, acute management is typically a recommendation of rest without medical intervention. Despite this, patients with mild TBI often exhibit significant disturbances in physical function, cognition, mood, and sleep quality.[37] In a normal course of recovery, most symptoms have resolved by the first week post-injury and patients are typically "back to normal" within 1 month post-injury,[60] but ~10% to 25% of patients fail to recover on this timeline and experience ongoing symptoms months to years after

injury.[38,39] Persistent symptoms are often given a label of post-concussion syndrome (PCS) based on clinical examination, medical history, and exercise tolerance tests.[61] Guidelines caution that PCS may not stem from a single pathophysiologic entity, but rather a variety of psychological and physiological factors.[37,62] The lack of clear unambiguous criteria limits the ability of physicians to diagnose, predict outcome, and develop treatments for patients with persistent symptoms.

One issue limiting research aimed in this area is that PCS encompasses heterogeneous clinical presentations and trajectories of recovery.[63,64] There is growing recognition that this heterogeneity likely originates from differences in the mechanisms of injury and subsequent adaptation.[65] Different symptom profiles (ie, predominantly somatic, cognitive, mood, or sleep-related) are thought to correspond to distinct "subtypes" of PCS with different recommended approaches to patient management.[62] Most definitions of PCS subtypes, however, are primarily based on clinical assessment at present[65] with more limited empirical support for underlying differences in neurophysiology.

In this respect, there is growing evidence that altered perfusion plays a role in post-concussion symptoms throughout the recovery process. Studies have indicated that lower frontal CBF within the first week of injury is associated with greater symptom severity and longer time to symptom resolution,[33] with similar relationships seen in the insular cortex at 1 month post-injury.[34] Conversely, other studies have found that higher posterior CBF is associated with more severe symptoms in the first week of injury[66] and at 1 month post-injury.[67] It is currently unknown whether the latter findings are also due to persistent CBF dysregulation or represent compensatory response to injury. Intriguingly, one ASL study found evidence that different symptom subtypes correlate with distinct patterns of CBF response,[66] as disturbances in posterior CBF were correlated with predominantly somatic complaints, whereas abnormal frontal CBF was related to predominantly cognitive complaints. A study of mild TBI conducted an average of 2 years post-injury also found that decreased thalamic CBF was correlated with worse neurocognitive outcomes, including processing and response speed, memory and learning, verbal fluency, and executive function.[68] Overall, these findings provide encouraging evidence of perfusion imaging as a biomarker for PCS and a potential target for interventions (Fig. 2). Further work is needed, however, to evaluate and characterize CBF effects within a more rigorous prognostic framework, before it can be integrated into clinical practice.

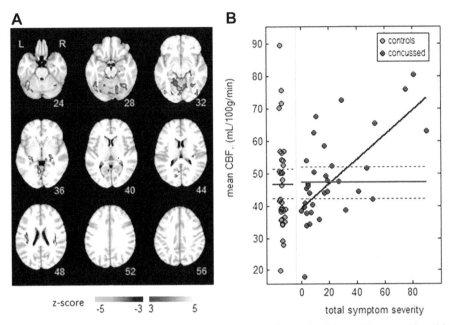

Fig. 2. Positive association of posterior CBF with acute symptoms, shown for 27 participants with mild TBI. CBF is regressed against total severity score on the sport concussion assessment tool (SCAT) with (*A*) significant brain regions identified and (*B*) mean regional values plotted against syptom severity scores, with a group of 27 controls for comparison. For the latter panel, the mean CBF values are plotted for control and mild TBI groups (black and red solid horizontal lines) along with 95% confidence bounds (dashed black and red lines). For the TBI group, the line of best fit regressing CBF onto symptoms is also plotted (angled black line). (*From* Churchill NW, Hutchison MG, Graham SJ, Schweizer TA. Symptom correlates of cerebral blood flow following acute concussion. Neuroimage Clin. 2017;16:234-239. Published 2017 Jul 24.)

SPORT CONCUSSION AND SAFE RETURN TO PLAY

The determination of "safe" return to activities is a major concern in the management of TBI across the severity spectrum. This has been most rigorously addressed in the sport setting, where it is established that premature return to sport will likely result in reinjury. In fact, a key predictor of concussion is having a prior history of concussion, which elevates both short-term and long-term risk of future injury.[69,70] Repeated mild TBIs also increase the risk of persistent cognitive deficits and noncognitive symptoms such as headaches, functional difficulties, and emotional disturbances,[71–73] significantly reducing quality of life. Clinical indices have been historically used to assess recovery, with epidemiological evidence used to refine minimum "stand-down" times. At present, consensus guidelines advocate for a graded exertional protocol, where athletes must first be asymptomatic at rest and then perform

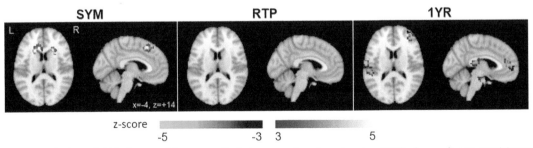

Fig. 3. Resolution of CBF abnormalities at medical clearance to return to play (RTP), shown for 24 participants with mild TBI, compared to a cohort of 122 controls. Significantly affected regions are shown for early symptomatic injury (SYM), RTP and one year post-RTP (1 YR). The early CBF abnormalities seen at SYM appear to be resolved at RTP, although new effects have emerged at 1 YR follow-up. (*From* Churchill NW, Hutchison MG, Graham SJ, Schweizer TA. Mapping brain recovery after concussion: From acute injury to 1 year after medical clearance. Neurology. 2019;93(21):e1980-e1992.)

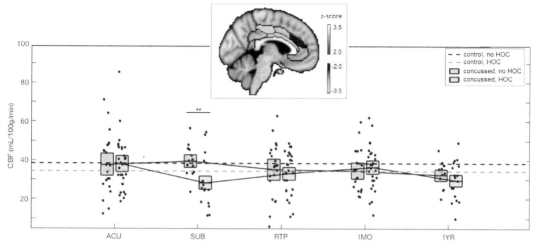

Fig. 4. Effects of prior history of concussion (HOC) on CBF in the cingulate cortex, shown for 67 participants with mild TBI, compared to a cohort of 167 controls. Significantly affected regions are shown (inset), and mean CBF is plotted with and without HOC, at acute and subacute injury (ACU, SUB), medical clearance to return to play (RTP), and 1 month and 1 year afterwards (1MO, 1 YR). Significantly greater CBF reductions are seen at SUB for individuals with prior HOC, as indicated by a '**' symbol. (*From* Churchill NW, Hutchison MG, Graham SJ, Schweizer TA. Acute and Chronic Effects of Multiple Concussions on Midline Brain Structures [published online ahead of print, 2021 Aug 25]. Neurology. 2021;97(12):e1170-e1181.)

increasingly strenuous activities without symptom onset. This symptom-oriented approach is advantageous, as it is straightforward to implement and it is directly tied to an athlete's ability to perform in the sport environment.

However, symptom assessments may be insensitive to subtle neural dysfunction and aspects of incomplete biological recovery that put individuals at risk of reinjury. Perfusion imaging is relevant, as the sensitivity of the cerebrovascular system may provide a probe of how long, and to what degree, brain function is disrupted post-injury. In terms of longitudinal recovery, the ASL literature indicates a rapidly evolving time course of recovery for CBF. As noted in Section "Effects of traumatic brain injury on perfusion," effects within the first week of injury are heterogeneous, with perfusion decreases often seen at the end of the week,[35,74] when most individuals are still symptomatic. A landmark study imaged concussed athletes 1 day, 1 week, and 1 month post-injury[34] and reported focal reductions in CBF of the insular and superior temporal cortex at 1 day, with normalization between 1 week and 1 month post-injury. This timeline followed the resolution of cognitive and neuropsychiatric symptoms. More recently, a longitudinal study similarly found that acute abnormalities in frontal CBF had dissipated at medical clearance, which occured at a median of 27 days post-injury[40] (Fig. 3). Such findings suggest that acute disturbances in resting CBF tend to normalize in concordance with standard symptom, balance, and cognitive metrics of recovery. One proviso, however, is that resting CBF may not provide a complete picture of recovery.

In the same manner that clinical guidelines emphasize the importance of testing symptoms under exertional load,[37] it has been suggested that neuroimaging combined with stress testing may expose functional deficits that are not detectable at rest.[75] In the perfusion domain, this is corroborated by a functional MR imaging study that examined cerebrovascular reactivity (CVR) during a breath-holding task.[76] This was measured longitudinally in concussed athletes, although the greatest disturbances were seen acutely, subtle changes in CVR continued up to 1 year after medical clearance to return to play. There is also evidence that repeated mild TBI may exacerbate and prolong post-concussion changes in CBF[77] (Fig. 4), potentially contributing to an increased risk of long-term neurodegenerative processes in the brain.[78] These results highlight the need to integrate perfusion imaging into clinical management and validate presumed recovery with comprehensive long-term follow-up.

SUMMARY

Cerebral perfusion is a tightly regulated component of neurophysiology and it is vulnerable to the effects of TBI across the severity spectrum. Perfusion imaging encompasses numerous CT and MR imaging techniques that can measure post-TBI changes in CBF. As discussed in this article, perfusion imaging provides a powerful approach for investigating complex changes in neurophysiology that occur after TBI in relation to clinical outcomes. Despite its substantial promise, this technology is underused in clinical practice and represents an important area of ongoing research. It is anticipated that the rapid pace of research, combined with refinement of existing imaging techniques, may accelerate the discovery process. Thus, we hope that perfusion imaging will soon provide new advances in evidence-based diagnosis and management of patients who suffer from TBI.

CLINICS CARE POINTS

- perfusion imaging has identified associations between cerebral blood flow (CBF) and outcome after traumatic brain injury (TBI), across the injury severity spectrum
- lower acute CBF values tend to predict poorer clinical outcome after a moderate-to-severe TBI
- reduced frontal and subcortical CBF are associated with more severe post-concussion symptoms
- CBF abnormalities tend to normalize concurrently with clinical metrics of recovery for sport-related concussion
- interpretations should be made cautiously, given the substantial heterogeneity in study methodologies and findings
- further large-scale prospective studies are needed before perfusion imaging can be fully integrated into clinical management of TBI

ACKNOWLEDGMENTS

This work was supported by the Canadian Institutes of Health Research (CIHR) [grant numbers RN356342 – 401065, RN294001–367456]; the Canadian Institute for Military and Veterans Health Research (CIMVHR) [grant number W7714-145967]; and Siemens Healthineers Canada.

DISCLOSURE

The authors have nothing to disclose.

REFERENCES

1. Thurman D, Guerrero J. Trends in hospitalization associated with traumatic brain injury. JAMA 1999; 282(10):954–7.

2. Len T, Neary J. Cerebrovascular pathophysiology following mild traumatic brain injury. Clin Physiol Funct Imaging 2011;31(2):85–93.

3. Malec JF, Brown AW, Leibson CL, et al. The mayo classification system for traumatic brain injury severity. J Neurotrauma 2007;24(9):1417–24.

4. Latchaw RE, Yonas H, Hunter GJ, et al. Guidelines and recommendations for perfusion imaging in cerebral ischemia: a scientific statement for healthcare professionals by the writing group on perfusion imaging, from the Council on Cardiovascular Radiology of the American Heart Association. Stroke 2003;34(4):1084–104.

5. Cunningham A, Salvador R, Coles J, et al. Physiological thresholds for irreversible tissue damage in contusional regions following traumatic brain injury. Brain 2005;128(8):1931–42.

6. Chan K-H, Miller JD, Piper IR. Cerebral blood flow at constant cerebral perfusion pressure but changing arterial and intracranial pressure: relationship to autoregulation. J Neurosurg Anesthesiol 1992;4(3):188–93.

7. Armstead WM. Cerebral blood flow autoregulation and dysautoregulation. Anesthesiology Clin 2016; 34(3):465–77.

8. Enevoldsen EM, Cold G, Jensen FT, et al. Dynamic changes in regional CBF, intraventricular pressure, CSF pH and lactate levels during the acute phase of head injury. J Neurosurg 1976; 44(2):191–214.

9. Jaggi JL, Obrist WD, Gennarelli TA, et al. Relationship of early cerebral blood flow and metabolism to outcome in acute head injury. J Neurosurg 1990; 72(2):176–82.

10. Maas AI, Stocchetti N, Bullock R. Moderate and severe traumatic brain injury in adults. Lancet Neurol 2008;7(8):728–41.

11. Prins M, Greco T, Alexander D, et al. The pathophysiology of traumatic brain injury at a glance. Dis Models Mech 2013;6(6):1307–15.

12. Werner C, Engelhard K. Pathophysiology of traumatic brain injury. Br J Anaesth 2007;99(1):4–9.

13. Robertson CS. Management of cerebral perfusion pressure after traumatic brain injury. J Am Soc Anesthesiologists 2001;95(6):1513–7.

14. Kinoshita K. Traumatic brain injury: pathophysiology for neurocritical care. J Intensive Care 2016;4(1):1–10.

15. Barzó P, Marmarou A, Fatouros P, et al. Contribution of vasogenic and cellular edema to traumatic brain swelling measured by diffusion-weighted imaging. J Neurosurg 1997;87(6):900–7.

16. Toklu HZ, Tumer N. Oxidative stress, brain edema, blood-brain barrier permeability, and autonomic dysfunction from traumatic brain injury. In: Kobeissy FH, editor. Brain Neurotrauma: Molecular, Neuropsychological, and Rehabilitation aspects. Boca Raton (FL): CRC Press/Taylor & Francis; 2015. p. 85–107.

17. Celli P, Fruin A, Cervoni L. Severe head trauma. Review of the factors influencing the prognosis. Minerva chirurgica 1997;52(12):1467–80.

18. Smith DH, Johnson VE, Stewart W. Chronic neuropathologies of single and repetitive TBI: substrates of dementia? Nat Rev Neurol 2013;9(4):211.

19. Smith M. Monitoring intracranial pressure in traumatic brain injury. Anesth Analgesia 2008;106(1): 240–8.

20. Schröder ML, Muizelaar JP, Bullock MR, et al. Focal ischemia due to traumatic contusions documented by stable xenon-CT and ultrastructural studies. J Neurosurg 1995;82(6):966–71.

21. Bouma GJ, Muizelaar JP, Stringer WA, et al. Ultra-early evaluation of regional cerebral blood flow in severely head-injured patients using xenon-enhanced computerized tomography. J Neurosurg 1992;77(3):360–8.

22. Marion DW, Darby J, Yonas H. Acute regional cerebral blood flow changes caused by severe head injuries. J Neurosurg 1991;74(3):407–14.

23. Corte FD, Giordano A, Pennisi M, et al. Quantitative cerebral blood flow and metabolism determination in the first 48 hours after severe head injury with a new dynamic SPECT device. Acta Neurochirurgica 1997; 139(7):636–42.

24. Inoue Y, Shiozaki T, Tasaki O, et al. Changes in cerebral blood flow from the acute to the chronic phase of severe head injury. J Neurotrauma 2005;22(12): 1411–8.

25. Yamakami I, McIntosh TK. Effects of traumatic brain injury on regional cerebral blood flow in rats as measured with radiolabeled microspheres. J Cereb Blood Flow Metab 1989;9(1):117–24.

26. Yuan X-Q, Prough DS, Smith TL, et al. The effects of traumatic brain injury on regional cerebral blood flow in rats. J Neurotrauma 1988;5(4):289–301.

27. Ginsberg M, Zhao W, Alonso O, et al. Uncoupling of local cerebral glucose metabolism and blood flow after acute fluid-percussion injury in rats. Am J Physiology-Heart Circulatory Physiol 1997;272(6): H2859–68.

28. Wang CX, Shuaib A. Critical role of microvasculature basal lamina in ischemic brain injury. Prog Neurobiol 2007;83(3):140–8.

29. Abdul-Muneer P, Schuetz H, Wang F, et al. Induction of oxidative and nitrosative damage leads to cerebrovascular inflammation in an animal model of mild traumatic brain injury induced by primary blast. Free Radic Biol Med 2013;60:282–91.

30. Truettner JS, Alonso OF, Dietrich WD. Influence of therapeutic hypothermia on matrix metalloproteinase activity after traumatic brain injury in rats. J Cereb Blood Flow Metab 2005;25(11):1505–16.

31. Strebel S, Lam AM, Matta BF, et al. Impaired cerebral autoregulation after mild brain injury. Surg Neurol 1997;47(2):128–31.

32. Giza CC, Hovda DA. The neurometabolic cascade of concussion. J Athletic Train 2001;36(3):228.

33. Churchill NW, Hutchison MG, Graham SJ, et al. Mapping recovery of brain physiology after concussion: from acute injury to one year after medical clearance. Neurology 2019;93(21):e1980–92.

34. Meier TB, Bellgowan PS, Singh R, et al. Recovery of cerebral blood flow following sports-related concussion. JAMA Neurol 2015;72(5):530–8.

35. Churchill NW, Hutchison MG, Richards D, et al. The first week after concussion: blood flow, brain function and white matter microstructure. NeuroImage: Clin 2017;14:480–9.

36. Giza CC, Hovda DA. The new neurometabolic cascade of concussion. Neurosurgery 2014; 75(suppl_4):S24–33.

37. McCrory P, Meeuwisse W, Dvorak J, et al. Consensus statement on concussion in sport—the 5th international conference on concussion in sport held in Berlin, October 2016. Br J Sports Med 2017;51(11):838–47.

38. CDC CfDCaP. Heads up: facts for physicians about mild traumatic brain injury. Atlanta, Georgia:CDC: MTBI); 2010.

39. Polinder S, Cnossen MC, Real RG, et al. A multidimensional approach to post-concussion symptoms in mild traumatic brain injury. Front Neurol 2018;9:1113.

40. Churchill NW, Hutchison MG, Graham SJ, et al. Mapping brain recovery after concussion: from acute injury to one year after medical clearance. Neurology 2019;93(21):e1980–92.

41. Yonas H, Pindzola RR, Johnson DW. Xenon/ computed tomography cerebral blood flow and its use in clinical management. Neurosurg Clin N Am 1996;7(4):605–16.

42. Grafton ST. PET: activation of cerebral blood flow and glucose metabolism. Adv Neurol 2000;83: 87–103.

43. Devous Sr MD. SPECT Functional Brain Imaging; Technical Considerations. J Neuroimaging 1995; 5(s1):s2–13.

44. Eastwood JD, Lev MH, Provenzale JM. Perfusion CT with iodinated contrast material. Am J Roentgenol 2003;180(1):3–12.

45. Koenig M, Kraus M, Theek C, et al. Quantitative assessment of the ischemic brain by means of perfusion-related parameters derived from perfusion CT. Stroke 2001;32(2):431–7.

46. Hunter GJ, Silvennoinen HM, Hamberg LM, et al. Whole-brain CT perfusion measurement of perfused cerebral blood volume in acute ischemic stroke: probability curve for regional infarction. Radiology 2003;227(3):725–30.

47. Østergaard L. Principles of cerebral perfusion imaging by bolus tracking. J Magn Reson Imaging 2005; 22(6):710–7.

48. Tofts PS, Kermode AG. Measurement of the blood-brain barrier permeability and leakage space using dynamic MR imaging. 1. Fundamental concepts. Magn Reson Med 1991;17(2):357–67.

49. Hackländer T, Reichenbach JR, Hofer M, et al. Measurement of cerebral blood volume via the relaxing effect of low-dose gadopentetate dimeglumine during bolus transit. Am J Neuroradiology 1996;17(5): 821–30.

50. Ferré J-C, Bannier E, Raoult H, et al. Arterial spin labeling (ASL) perfusion: techniques and clinical use. Diagn Interv Imaging 2013;94(12):1211–23.

51. Alsop DC, Detre JA, Golay X, et al. Recommended implementation of arterial spin-labeled perfusion MRI for clinical applications: a consensus of the ISMRM perfusion study group and the European consortium for ASL in dementia. Magn Reson Med 2015;73(1):102–16.

52. Pollock JM, Tan H, Kraft RA, et al. Arterial spin-labeled MR perfusion imaging: clinical applications. Magn Reson Imaging Clin N Am 2009;17(2):315–38.

53. Vella MA, Crandall ML, Patel MB. Acute management of traumatic brain injury. Surg Clin 2017; 97(5):1015–30.

54. Wintermark M, Van Melle G, Schnyder P, et al. Admission perfusion CT: prognostic value in patients with severe head trauma. Radiology 2004;232(1):211–20.

55. Kaloostian P, Robertson C, Gopinath SP, et al. Outcome prediction within twelve hours after severe traumatic brain injury by quantitative cerebral blood flow. J Neurotrauma 2012;29(5):727–34.

56. Fridley J, Robertson C, Gopinath S. Quantitative lobar cerebral blood flow for outcome prediction after traumatic brain injury. J Neurotrauma 2015;32(2):75–82.

57. Honda M, Ichibayashi R, Yokomuro H, et al. Early cerebral circulation disturbance in patients suffering from severe traumatic brain injury (TBI): a xenon CT and perfusion CT study. Neurologia Medico-chirurgica 2016;56(8):501–9.

58. Shankar JJS, Green R, Virani K, et al. Admission perfusion CT for classifying early in-hospital mortality of patients with severe traumatic brain injury: a pilot study. Am J Roentgenol 2020;214(4):872–6.

59. Soustiel JF, Mahamid E, Goldsher D, et al. Perfusion-CT for early assessment of traumatic cerebral contusions. Neuroradiology 2008;50(2):189–96.

60. Foundation ON. Guidelines for concussion/mild traumatic brain injury & persistent symptoms: for adults (18+ years of age). Ottawa, Ontario: Ontario Neurotrauma Foundation; 2013.

61. Ellis MJ, Leddy JJ, Willer B. Physiological, vestibulo-ocular and cervicogenic post-concussion disorders: an evidence-based classification system with directions for treatment. Brain Inj 2015;29(2):238–48.

62. Leddy JJ, Sandhu H, Sodhi V, et al. Rehabilitation of concussion and post-concussion syndrome. Sports Health 2012;4(2):147–54.

63. Lingsma HF, Roozenbeek B, Steyerberg EW, et al. Early prognosis in traumatic brain injury: from prophecies to predictions. Lancet Neurol 2010;9(5): 543–54.

64. Hiploylee C, Dufort PA, Davis HS, et al. Longitudinal study of postconcussion syndrome: not everyone recovers. J Neurotrauma 2017;34(8):1511–23.

65. Rosenbaum SB, Lipton ML. Embracing chaos: the scope and importance of clinical and pathological heterogeneity in mTBI. Brain Imaging Behav 2012; 6(2):255–82.

66. Churchill NW, Hutchison MG, Graham SJ, et al. Symptom correlates of cerebral blood flow following acute concussion. Neuroimage: Clin 2017;16:234–9.

67. Lin C-M, Tseng Y-C, Hsu H-L, et al. Arterial spin labeling perfusion study in the patients with subacute mild traumatic brain injury. PLoS One 2016;11(2): e0149109.

68. Ge Y, Patel MB, Chen Q, et al. Assessment of thalamic perfusion in patients with mild traumatic brain injury by true FISP arterial spin labelling MR imaging at 3T. Brain Inj 2009;23(7–8):666–74.

69. Guskiewicz KM, McCrea M, Marshall SW, et al. Cumulative effects associated with recurrent concussion in collegiate football players: the NCAA Concussion Study. JAMA 2003;290(19):2549–55.

70. Iverson GL, Gaetz M, Lovell MR, et al. Cumulative effects of concussion in amateur athletes. Brain Inj 2004;18(5):433–43.

71. Guskiewicz KM, Marshall SW, Bailes J, et al. Association between recurrent concussion and late-life cognitive impairment in retired professional football players. Neurosurgery 2005;57(4):719–26.

72. Guskiewicz KM, Marshall SW, Bailes J, et al. Recurrent concussion and risk of depression in retired professional football players. Med Sci Sports Exerc 2007;39(6):903.

73. Ryan LM, Warden DL. Post concussion syndrome. Int Rev Psychiatry 2003;15(4):310–6.

74. Wang Y, Nelson LD, LaRoche AA, et al. Cerebral blood flow alterations in acute sport-related concussion. J Neurotrauma 2016;33(13):1227–36.

75. Zhang K, Johnson B, Gay M, et al. Default mode network in concussed individuals in response to the YMCA physical stress test. J Neurotrauma 2012;29(5):756–65.

76. Churchill N, Hutchison M, Graham S, et al. Cerebrovascular reactivity after sport concussion: from acute injury to one year after medical clearance. Front Neurol 2020;11:558.

77. Churchill NW, Hutchison MG, Graham SJ, et al. Acute and chronic effects of multiple concussions on midline brain structures. Neurology 2021; 97(12):e1170–81.

78. Gavett BE, Stern RA, Cantu RC, et al. Mild traumatic brain injury: a risk factor for neurodegeneration. Alzheimer's Res Ther 2010;2(3):18.

Traumatic Brain Injury and Vision

Mary D. Maher, MD[a], Mohit Agarwal, MD[b], Madhura A. Tamhankar, MD[c], Suyash Mohan, MD, PDCC[a,d],*

KEYWORDS

- Cranial nerve • Afferent pathway • Efferent pathway • Visual pathways

KEY POINTS

- Review of visual symptoms in patients with traumatic brain injury.
- Review of the afferent and efferent visual pathways.
- Review of imaging techniques for injury to visual pathways.

MAIN TEXT

An astounding 70% of sensory processing is affected by vision,[1] and 40% of the brain serves the primarily visual function.[2] Cranial nerves II, III, IV, V, VI, and VII are involved with the visual system along with the parasympathetic and sympathetic fibers of the autonomic system. Cranial nerve II is the optic nerve. Cranial nerve III is the oculomotor nerve, which innervates the medial rectus, inferior rectus, inferior oblique, superior rectus, and levator palpebrae superioris muscles. Cranial nerve IV is the trochlear nerve, which innervates the superior oblique muscle. Cranial nerve V is the trigeminal nerve, which provides sensory innervation. Cranial nerve VI is the abducens nerve, which innervates the lateral rectus muscle. Cranial nerve VII is the facial nerve, which innervates the orbicularis oculi muscle. The autonomic parasympathetic fibers travel along the periphery of the oculomotor nerve, innervating the sphincter pupillae muscle to constrict the pupil and innervate the ciliary muscles to alter the shape of the lens for convergence. Autonomic sympathetic fibers innervate the dilator pupillae muscle which dilates the pupil.[3] The complex and widespread anatomic distribution of the optic pathway, as well as the primary visual cortex and secondary visual processing centers can be involved by the diffuse nature of traumatic brain injury (TBI) at multiple sites and the array of resulting visual complaints can be multitudinous. Understanding the anatomy of the visual pathway is therefore critical to understand the visual symptoms following TBI.

The pathophysiology of TBI can be divided into primary and secondary injuries. *Primary* injury results from direct mechanical forces,[4] whereas *secondary* injury may begin immediately after the trauma but has a more prolonged course in the form of a cascade of cellular and tissue response to injury, involving oxidative stress, inflammatory mediators, blood–brain barrier breakdown, increased macrophage activity, and, ultimately, excitotoxic damage and cellular apoptosis.[5] This twofold mechanism of injury in TBI is applicable to all of the central nervous system circuitry, including the visual pathways.

The visual system can be divided into afferent and efferent pathways. Within these pathways, the primary and secondary injuries of TBI cause visual loss and ocular motor dysfunction. Visual

[a] Division of Neuroradiology, Department of Radiology, Perelman School of Medicine at the University of Pennsylvania, 3400 Spruce Street, Philadelphia, PA 19104, USA; [b] Division of Neuroradiology, Department of Radiology, Medical College of Wisconsin, 9200 W Wisconsin Avenue, Milwaukee, WI 53226, USA; [c] Division of Neuro-Ophthalmology, Department of Ophthalmology, Perelman School of Medicine at the University of Pennsylvania, 3400 Spruce Street, Philadelphia, PA 19104, USA; [d] Department of Neurosurgery, Perelman School of Medicine at the University of Pennsylvania, 3400 Spruce Street, Philadelphia, PA 19104, USA
* Corresponding author. Division of NeuroradiologyDepartment of RadiologyPerelman School of Medicine at the University of Pennsylvania 3400 Spruce Street, Philadelphia, PA 19104.
E-mail address: suyash.mohan@pennmedicine.upenn.edu

Neuroimag Clin N Am 33 (2023) 325–333
https://doi.org/10.1016/j.nic.2023.01.007

symptoms of mild TBI include photophobia, accommodative dysfunction (convergence insufficiency or convergence spasm), and saccadic and/or pursuit dysfunction. TBI is most commonly seen and studied in the military and sports-related injuries in the civilian population. In a young cohort of patients between 11 and 17 years of age with mild TBI, the visual symptoms were accommodative dysfunction (51%) and saccadic dysfunction (29%).[2] In a Veterans Health Administration (VA) clinic dedicated to visual problems of polytrauma survivors, photophobia was the most common complaint (55%) followed by near vision dysfunction, including accommodating insufficiency (23%), all of which were increased in the setting of loss of consciousness associated with the TBI.[6]

The Afferent Visual Pathway

Photophobia is one of the most common visual symptoms following mild TBI and is related to a dysfunctional afferent sensory system. Hypersensitivity to light is regulated through the trigeminal sensory system. Melanopsinergic intrinsically photosensitive retinal ganglion cells (ipRGC) and the cornea and iris have been hypothesized to stimulate the nociceptive trigeminothalamic pathway and sensory cortex.[4] The ipRGC cells project to the suprachiasmatic nucleus, affecting circadian rhythm; the Edinger-Westphal nucleus, affecting pupillary response; and the thalamus, affecting the pain centers.[7] Though the ipRGC population of cells accounts for 0.2% to 0.8% of ganglion cells, they are disproportionately able to survive the injury.[7] Photophobia is highest in the first week after TBI (30.46%) with a steady decline until three months (13.51%) and continues to decrease in the chronic phase in civilians. Military veterans experience more severe and prolonged photophobia than the civilian population which is hypothesized to be related to the diffuse nature of blast injuries rather than focal sport or other civilian injuries.[8] Within the cohort of veterans with TBI, women experience greater photophobia than men.[9] Functional MRI (fMRI) has demonstrated the intersection of afferent visual processing with nociceptive trigeminal pathways by showing pulvinar activation during melanopsinergic ipRGC stimulation in a patient with idiopathic photophobia.[4,10] A perfusion single-photon emission computerized tomography study of patients with mild or moderate TBI showed that hypoperfusion was greatest in the basal ganglia, and most common in the thalami followed by frontal and temporal lobes.[11]

The afferent visual pathway transmits light from the retina through the optic nerve, chiasm, optic tracts, lateral geniculate ganglion, and optic radiations to the primary visual cortex.[12,13] Damage to these structures causes vision loss and/or visual field deficits. Direct trauma to the eye can damage a myriad of orbital and ocular structures, causing lid lacerations, globe rupture (Fig. 1) with retinochoroidal injury, and traumatic optic neuropathy. TBI can cause indirect damage to the optic nerve, optic chiasm, optic tract, optic radiations, and the occipital lobe.[14]

Traumatic optic neuropathy can result from direct penetrating injury or indirect injury to the optic nerve such as avulsion injury, stretch injury, shearing, contusion, or compression.[15] The small, confined space of the optic nerve canal is particularly vulnerable to direct injury by adjacent fractures or intracranial pressure shifts.[5,15] Recovery from direct optic neuropathy is uncommon and surgical intervention is often unsuccessful in restoring vision.[5,15] Eye trauma causing retrobulbar hematoma can also cause an acute increase in the intraocular pressure and decrease perfusion with variable vision loss (Fig. 2).[15] In the acute setting, a head computed tomography (CT) head can reveal a displaced intracanalicular fracture (Fig. 3), optic nerve sheath, or retrobulbar

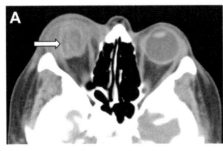
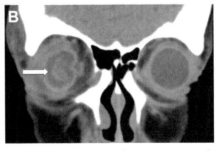

Fig. 1. Right monocular vision loss after a fall presented with right eye pain, no light perception in the right eye. Axial (*A*) and coronal (*B*) head CT without contrast demonstrates right globe rupture with a large right retinal tear (*arrows*), detectable on the CT without contrast. Reproduced, with permission, from Maher M, et al. Imaging Acute Ophthalmic Trauma. American Academy of Ophthalmology. Available at: https://www.aao.org/course/imaging-acute-ocular-trauma. Accessed Sept. 11, 2022.

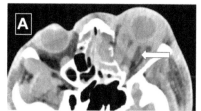
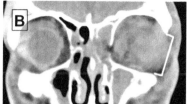
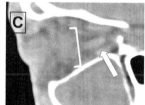

Fig. 2. Left monocular vision loss after altercation. Left medial wall fracture resulting in optic nerve injury with optic nerve thickening (*arrow* in *A* and *C*) and retrobulbar hemorrhage (*bracket* in *B* and *C*) and proptosis. The patient required an emergency lateral canthotomy and inferior cantholysis to decrease the high intra-orbital pressure and preserve vision. Reproduced, with permission, from Maher M, et al. Imaging Acute Ophthalmic Trauma. American Academy of Ophthalmology. Available at: https://www.aao.org/course/imaging-acute-ocular-trauma. Accessed Sept. 11, 2022.

hematoma. Decompressive canthotomy and cantholysis often need to be performed emergently to decrease the intraocular pressure and prevent vision loss due to optic neuropathy that can ensue if it is untreated.

Indirect traumatic optic neuropathy arises from either propagation of blunt impact stress waves through the bone to the intracanalicular optic nerve or pulling of the optic nerve in a coup countercoup head injury and can occur in the setting of even mild trauma[5,16] It often results from injury to the forehead that causes transmission of forces through the intracanalicular segment of the bone causing shearing and disruption of the blood supply to the optic nerve via the pial plexus. Vision loss may be immediate or may occur over the course of several days, likely from optic nerve ischemia.[5]

Diffusion tensor imaging (DTI) or diffusion tensor tractography (DTT) measures the preferential direction of water diffusion and can indicate optic nerve injury. Water diffusion has directionality along the axon, called anisotropy, which is measured by fractional anisotropy (FA).[17] Axial diffusivity (AD) refers to the diffusion of water along or parallel to axons. Radial diffusivity (RD) is diffusion perpendicular to axons.[17] Mean diffusivity (MD) accounts for diffusivities in all directions and is overall decreased in acute injury in the setting of cytotoxic edema.[17] When there is a loss of axonal integrity after injury, there is loss of directionality (loss of anisotropy).[17] FA decreases due to the loss of direction-oriented diffusion of water along damaged axons.

DTI has revealed decreased FA in the optic nerve between 7 and 30 days after indirect traumatic optic neuropathy.[18] The cohort greater than 30 days from injury demonstrated decreased FA, decreased AD, increased RD, and increased MD.[18] The decrease in FA values corresponded to decreasing retinal nerve fiber layer (RNFL) and ganglion cell complex (GCC) in the macula.[18] The decrease in MD and AD is greatest in the posterior segment of the optic nerve, supporting evidence that axonal damage is greatest at the optic canal, leading to axonal swelling.[17] At autopsy, hemorrhage, demyelination, focal necrosis, and axonal damage were identified, suggesting

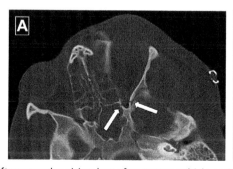
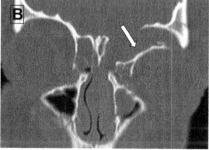

Fig. 3. Left monocular vision loss after motor vehicle accident. (A) CT without contrast shows a fracture that extends through the orbital apex (*arrow*) without displacement of a fracture fragment into the apex. (B) CT without contrast shows a right orbital roof and medial orbital wall fracture with displacement of the fracture fragment into the orbit (*arrow*). Reproduced, with permission, from Maher M, et al. Imaging Acute Ophthalmic Trauma. American Academy of Ophthalmology. Available at: https://www.aao.org/course/imaging-acute-ocular-trauma. Accessed Sept. 11, 2022.

vascular thrombosis or spasm may also be present[17,19]

In one patient with traumatic optic tract syndrome, atrophy of the left optic tract was identified on conventional MR imaging with decreased FA and increased MD on DTI.[20] In the patients with mild TBI and visual complaints but without abnormality on conventional MR imaging, mean FA values and tract volume of the optic radiations were significantly lower than controls.[21] Patients with chronic optic neuropathy from conditions such as multiple sclerosis have also shown decreased FA values in optic radiations, also reflecting antegrade trans-synaptic degeneration.[22] Decreased FA values are not specific for traumatic optic neuropathies as multiple sclerosis patients with chronic optic neuritis have also shown a decrease in FA in the prefrontal and temporal regions.[23]

As early as 1890, the visual cortex was localized to the occipital lobes, which specifically could produce a contralateral hemianopia. The lower visual field localizes to the upper bank of the calcarine fissure, and the upper visual field localizes to the lower calcarine fissure.[13] Central foveal vision localizes in a retinotopic map in the occipital poles with progressively eccentric peripheral vision localizing to the progressively anterior cortex along the calcarine fissure.[24]

Though the striate cortex (V1) is the primary visual cortex and the predominant output from the lateral geniculate ganglion, not all retinal input is signaled directly into the striate cortex.[13] There is output from the pulvinar and lateral geniculate ganglion that bypass the striate cortex to alternative cortices for processing.[13] For example, visual motion is processed by the middle temporal area (V5).[13] fMRI has identified six distinct visual areas in addition to striate cortex (V1).[13,24]

MR spectroscopy (MRS) examines metabolic activity and can be useful to measure neuronal injury and recovery. Measurable changes can be detected without the presence of neuronal death by this modality.[25] In post-concussive symptomatic patients, MRS detected decreased white matter N-acetylaspartate (NAA), a marker of neuronal integrity.[25] Decreased NAA is measured relative to creatine (Cr) and choline (Cho), which are markers of energy consumption and cell turnover, respectively. Decreased NAA levels and increased Cho levels were identified in regions of contusion evident on anatomic sequences from direct injury and even in regions of normal-appearing white matter on anatomic sequences, which may reflect underlying diffuse axonal injury or a component of Wallerian degeneration.[26] The NAA level recovers following injury although metabolite recovery can lag behind symptom resolution. In the setting of multiple episodes of mild TBI, normalization of NAA is delayed.[25]

Chemical exchange saturation transfer (CEST) is used to measure metabolite concentration, similar to MRS but with higher sensitivity and special resolution.[26] Glutamate is an excitatory neurotransmitter that is increased in the setting of TBI, which causes neurotoxicity and is quantifiable with CEST imaging. One study showed that small, though statistically significant, increases in glutamate were measured in the parieto-occipital white matter of patients with TBI and poor clinical outcomes, compared with patients with TBI and good clinical outcomes, as well as healthy control cohorts.[26]

Arterial spin labeling (ASL) allows the evaluation of perfusion by MR imaging using blood as an endogenous tracer. This technique has the advantages of no radiation, good spatial resolution, and minimal artifacts. Patients with mild TBI demonstrate lower cerebral blood flow (CBF) in the bifrontal and left occipital lobe in the subacute phase of injury which is hypothesized to be related to shearing forces of white matter at the thalamus and direct contact injury to the cortex.[27,28] Most studies have shown decreased CBF during the chronic phase of injury.[27] Interestingly, patients with more severe symptoms demonstrate increased CBF in these regions, which are not fully understood but perhaps related to altered cerebral hemodynamics.[27]

The Efferent Visual Pathway

The efferent visual pathway is involved with the coordination of eye movements to allow foveal fixation on the object of interest.[12] Central control of eye movements is initiated in the cerebral cortex and transmitted along the axons of the white matter. Some of these axons go directly to the cranial nerve nuclei III, IV, and VI within the brain stem, and others are routed through the superior colliculus (SC) of the tectum to map out the movements before going to cranial nerve nuclei in the brain stem. Complex interneurons that connect the cranial nerve nuclei and interact with nuclei in the brain stem and cerebellum are also involved in conjugate gaze horizontally and vertically. Coordinated eye movements require complex neuronal circuitry to be intact. Injury to any element results in ocular motor disturbances resulting in diplopia from ocular motor nerve paresis, disturbances in saccades and pursuits, accommodative dysfunction, or convergence insufficiency or spasm.

Mild TBIs that cause visual processing deficits are frequently related to abnormal coordination of the eye movements. The vast territory of gray and white matter involved in vision highlights how a diffuse injury such as mild TBI can affect the complex circuitry and connectivity of the visual system. Cortical control of vision involves the frontal eye field (FEF), the parietal eye field (PEF), the supplementary eye field (SEF), the dorsolateral prefrontal cortex, and the temporal cortex (area MT). The FEF is located in the vicinity of the precentral gyrus and the dorsal-most portion of the superior frontal sulcus and gives motor commands for the eye movements. The FEF releases the inhibitory control of the substantia nigra on the SC. With this disinhibition, the SC integrates motor commands from the FEF and visual attention from the intraparietal area of the posterior parietal cortex.[12] If the FEF is damaged (Fig. 4), there is a contralateral gaze palsy that recovers over time because the SC will adapt to respond to parietal stimulation alone. Likewise, if there is damage to the SC, saccade latency (moving eyes rapidly to a particular point in remembered space) is transient, because of the FEF fibers which project directly from the FEF to the brainstem nuclei remain intact. Damage to both the FEF and the SC result in a permanent deficit.[12]

The PEF is located in the posterior region of the intraparietal sulcus and is important for visual attention and saccades. A saccade is a rapid voluntary movement of both eyes to bring an object onto the fovea.[12] The two eyes are conjugate or coordinated in this movement. Saccades are the basis of reading, the memory guidance of bringing the eyes from the end of a line of text to the remembered point in space of the beginning of the next line.[2] Driving requires similar coordination. fMRI has demonstrated increased posterior parietal cortex stimulation during saccades. Damage to the PEF results in a latency of saccades, selective neglect and attentional deficits, and irregular smooth pursuit. Damage to the bilateral PEF affects the triggering of saccades.[12]

The SEF is located anterior to the supplementary motor area (SMA) in the superior paracentral sulcus and is essential in hand-eye coordination, motor control of successive saccades, and combined saccade and body motion.[12] The dorsolateral prefrontal cortex inhibits saccades in the setting of a higher-priority task.[12]

The temporal cortex (area MT) is located in the occipito-temporo-parietal junction, detects motion and is involved in the visual processing of motion, smooth pursuit, optokinetic nystagmus (OKN), and vestibulo-ocular reflex (VOR). Damage to MT impairs response to moving objects and smooth pursuit. In contrast to saccades which bring a steady object into focus with a rapidly moving gaze as seen in reading, smooth pursuit brings a moving object into focus on the fovea by

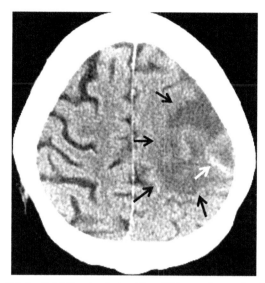

Fig. 4. Axial standard algorithm CT image in a patient with traumatic brain injury with right gaze palsy shows subarachnoid hemorrhage (*white arrow*) and cytotoxic edema (*black arrows*) in the left superior and middle frontal gyri/sulci. The cytotoxic edema involves the FEF. Lesions involving the FEFs cause gaze palsy such that the eyes deviate to the side of the lesion.

matching the velocity of the eye to the velocity of the moving object. The middle temporal area perceives the motion and velocity of the object and activates the FEF to command motion through the dorsolateral pontine nuclei to the cerebellar vermis and flocculus along the cortico-ponto-cerebellar pathway. fMRI can demonstrate abnormal activity on smooth pursuits testing without localization, suggesting a more global disruption of connectivity.[2]

OKN describes the phenomenon of following a large moving field of view. The eyes move slowly to watch the entire scene and quickly adjust when the scene is out of view. Both temporal and parietal lobes are critical in OKN, perceiving velocity and spatial processing, respectively. In contrast to saccades, smooth pursuit, and OKN in which the object or eyes are moving, VOR keeps the object of focus stable on the fovea while the head is moving. The VOR requires visual, vestibular, cerebellar, and motor integration and includes input from the visual cortex, the superior temporal sulcus, the occipito-temporal region, and posterior parietal cortex.[12]

Accommodation helps to focus the objects on the retina at different distances by changing the shape of the lens and is enabled by the contraction of the ciliary muscles. It is accompanied by convergence that involves contraction of the medial rectus muscles. The cortical region for

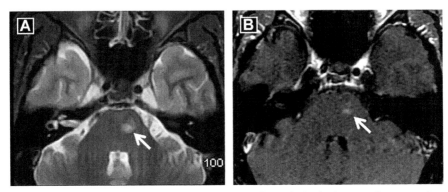

Fig. 5. Axial STIR (*A*) and T1+C fat suppressed (*B*) MR imaging through the brain stem show an enhancing active demyelinating lesion (*arrows*) in a patient with known multiple sclerosis who presented with left gaze palsy. Neural pathways subserving horizontal eye movements converge on the PPRF and lesions in this location cause gaze palsy with the eye deviating opposite to the side of the lesion. Hemorrhagic lesions in TBI can lead to similar horizontal gaze palsy.

convergence is the posterior parietal cortex, frontal cortex, and the preoccipital cortex. Left temporal lobe lesions can result in convergence paralysis, suggesting an additional region of cortical control.[12]

The oculomotor, trochlear, and abducens nerves are cranial nerves with motor nuclei in the brainstem that innervate the extraocular muscles. Normal eye movements are conjugate, meaning the extraocular muscles are simultaneously and symmetrically stimulated to achieve parallel movements of the eyes to bring objects onto the fovea, the center of vision. TBI can cause lesions involving the cranial nerve nuclei anywhere along their anatomic course from the brainstem to the orbit and may result in ocular motor deficits. These deficits may cause isolated ocular motor palsy or

paralysis of conjugate eye movements when internuclear pathways such as the medial longitudinal fasciculus (MLF), paramedian pontine reticular formation (PPRF), and rostral interstitial nucleus of medial longitudinal fasciculus (riMLF) are involved or gaze paresis from cortical involvement (**Figs. 5** and **6**).

The MLF is a bilateral white matter tract that runs parallel to the fourth ventricle in the brainstem which connects bilateral oculomotor, trochlear, and abducens nuclei for coordinated conjugate eye movements and carries vestibular signals for eye movement control. For example, when gazing to the left, the left lateral rectus is stimulated by the left abducens nerve to contract and pull the left globe laterally. Interneurons cross the midline from the left abducens nucleus and travel in the

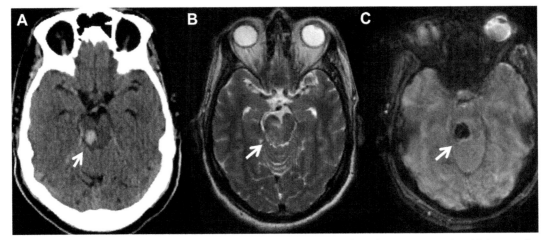

Fig. 6. Axial standard algorithm CT (*A*), axial T2W MR imaging (*B*) and axial SWI MR imaging (*C*) in a patient presenting with vertical gaze palsy. A hemorrhagic lesion is seen in the right midbrain (*arrows*). The vertical gaze centers (riMLF and the INC) are located in the midbrain and lesions in this location result in vertical gaze palsy.

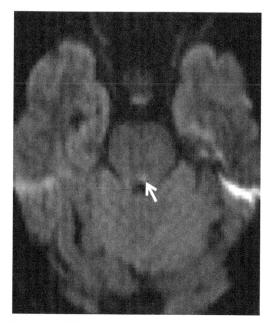

Fig. 7. Axial DWI MR imaging shows an infarct in the MLF (*arrow*) in a patient presenting with internuclear ophthalmoplegia and vertigo. The MLF is a bundle of white matter fibers that interconnects the cranial nerve III, IV, and V nuclei for conjugate eye movements and carries vestibular signals for eye movement control.

contralateral longitudinal fasciculus to stimulate the right oculomotor nerve to contract the right medial rectus to achieve conjugate eye movement. Damage to the MLF (Fig. 7) results in internuclear ophthalmoplegia with failure of adduction of the contralateral eye and dysconjugate gaze.[12]

The riMLF and the interstitial nucleus of Cajal (INC) within the MLF coordinate more complex input into coordinated eye movement. The riMLF is close to the oculomotor nuclei and essential to vertical saccades, connecting FEF, PEF, and SC, the oculomotor nuclei, and the cerebellum. Damage results in ipsilateral or bilateral loss of vertical saccades.[12] The INC within the MLF is adjacent to the riMLF and integrates commands to maintain gaze with vertical and torsional eye movements, connecting the contralateral INC through the posterior commissure, the oculomotor and trochlear nuclei, both MLF and the vestibular nuclei.[29] Bilateral INC damage results in impairment in eccentric gaze holding and vertical VOR; unilateral INC damage results in torsional nystagmus. Damage to the posterior commissure results in paralysis of upward gaze and convergence and can be associated with mydriasis, ptosis, and accommodative loss in Parinaud's syndrome.[12]

Several nuclei within the cerebellum are important for eye movements. The flocculus and paraflocculus at the inferior aspect of the cerebellum are part of the vestibulocochlear reflex, important in smooth pursuit and gaze holding. Damage to the flocculus will impair smooth pursuit and gaze holding, resulting in gaze-evoked nystagmus after eccentric eye movements and downbeat nystagmus in which the gaze cannot be held; the eyes drift away from eccentric gaze followed by a saccade to rapidly correct the drift. The fastigial nuclei within the superior vermis regulate saccades to ensure the gaze arrives on target. Damage to the fastigial nucleus results in saccadic hypermetria or hypometria, overshooting, or undershooting the target, respectively. Bilateral hypermetria results if both fastigial nuclei are damaged. The uvula and pyramidal vermis are important in the modulation of VOR, and damage of these results in deficits in smooth pursuits, and slow phases of OKN, and impairs the function of VOR. Damage to the nodulus and paravermal region results in periodic alternating nystagmus and horizontal jerk nystagmus with a change in direction.[12]

Visual symptoms of TBI involve both the afferent and efferent visual pathways. Because of the intricate anatomy of the visual system which is both complex and expansive, the diffuse nature of TBI has significant visual repercussions for injured patients. Our understanding of visual system connectivity and our ability to meaningfully image and interpret injury will continue to improve as imaging techniques evolve over time.

CLINICS CARE POINTS

- Injury to the *afferent* visual pathway results in vision and/or visual field loss from injury to the optic pathways and photophobia from injury to the nociceptive trigeminothalamic pathway and sensory cortex.

- Injury to the *efferent* visual pathway results in eye movement abnormalities causing ocular misalignment, nystagmus, saccadic and pursuit dysmetria, and accommodative insufficiency and can involve the frontal, parietal, and temporal cortex as well as white matter, brainstem, and cerebellum.

- Diffusion tensor imaging or diffusion tensor tractography is an important diagnostic tool that can assess injury to the afferent and efferent pathways.

FUNDING

The author(s) received no financial support for the research, authorship, and/or publication of this article.

CONFLICT OF INTEREST

The authors state that all authors do not have any potential conflicts of interest.

AUTHORSHIP

M.D. Maher: Main article drafting and revision. Figure contribution. M. Agarwal: Main article drafting and revision. Figure Contribution. M.A. Tamhanka: Main article drafting and revision. Figure contribution. S. Mohan: Main article drafting and revision. Figure contribution.

REFERENCES

1. Goodrich GL, Kirby J, Cockerham G, et al. Visual function in patients of a polytrauma rehabilitation center: a descriptive study. J Rehabil Res Dev 2007;44(7):929–36.
2. Singman EL, Quaid P. Vision disorders in mild traumatic brain injury. Neurosensory Disorders in Mild Traumatic Brain Injury. In: Michael E, editor. Hoffer and carey david balaban. Academic Press, an Imprint of Elsevier; 2019. p. 223–44.
3. Som PM, Curtin HD. Head and neck imaging. 5th ed. Mosby Elsevier; 2001.
4. Deil RJ, Mehra D, Kardon R, et al. Photophobia: shared pathophysiology underlying dry eye disease, migraine and traumatic brain injury leading to central neuroplasticity of the trigeminothalamic pathway. Br J Ophthalmol 2021;105(6):751–60.
5. Atkins EJ, Newman NJ, Biousse V. Post-traumatic visual loss. Rev Neurol Dis 2008;5(2):73–81.
6. Magone MT, Kwon E, Shin SY. Chronic visual dysfunction after blast-induced mild traumatic brain injury. J Rehabil Res Dev 2014;51(1):71–80.
7. Katz BJ, Digre KB. Diagnosis, pathophysiology and treatment of photophobia. Surv Ophthalmol 2016; 61(4):466–77.
8. Merezhibshkaya N, Mallia RK, Park D, et al. Photophobia Associated with Traumatic Brain Injury: A Systematic Review and Meta-analysis. Optom Vis Sci 2021;98(8):891–900.
9. Brickell TA, Lippa SM, French LM, et al. Female Service Members and Symptom Reporting after Combat and Non-Combat-Related Mild Traumatic Brain Injury. J Neurotrauma 2017;34(2):300–12. Epub 2016 Aug 5. PMID: 27368356.
10. Paorgias A, Lee D, Silva KE, et al. Blue light activates pulvinar nuclei in longstanding idiopathic photophobia: a case report. Neuroimage: Clinical 2019;24:102096.
11. Abdel-Dayem HM, Adu-Judeh H, Mithilesh K, et al. SPECT Brain Perfusion Abnormalities in Mild or Moderate Traumatic Brain Injury. Clin Nucl Med 1998;23(5):309–17.
12. Agarwal M, Ulmer JL, Chandra T, et al. Imaging correlates of neural control of ocular movements. Eur Radiol 2015;26(7):2193–205.
13. Zeki S, Leff A. The striate cortex and hemianopia. In: Barton JJS, Leff A, editors. Handbook of clinical neurology: neurology of vision and visual disorders, 3. Elsevier; 2021. p. 115–29. https://doi.org/10.1016/B978-0-12-821377-3.00004-0, 178.
14. Maher M., Woreta F., Auran J.D., et al., Imaging acute ophthalmic trauma. American Academy of Ophthalmology, Available at: https://www.aao.org/course/imaging-acute-ocular-trauma, 2020. Accessed February 16, 2022.
15. Ventura RE, Balcer LJ, Galetta SL. The neuro-ophthalmology of head trauma. Lancet Neurol 2014;13:1006–16.
16. Li Y, Singman E, McCulley T, et al. The biomechanics of indirect traumatic optic neuropathy using a computational head model with a biofidelic orbit. Front Neurol 2020;11:346.
17. Bodanapally UK, Kathirkamanathan S, Geraymovych E, et al. Diagnosis of traumatic optic neuropathy: application of diffusion tensor magnetic resonance imaging. J Neuro Ophthalmol 2013 Jun; 33(2):128–33.
18. Li J, Shi W, Li M, et al. Time-dependent diffusion tensor changes of optic nerve in patients with indirect traumatic optic neuropathy. Acta Radiologica 2014;55(7):855–63.
19. Cockerham KP. "Traumatic optic neuropathy." ophthalmic Care of the combat casualty. Edited by AB thach. Washington, DC: TMM Publications; 2003. p. 395–403.
20. Al-Zubidi N, Ansari W, Fung SH, et al. Diffusion Tensor Imaging in Traumatic Optic Tract Syndrome. J Neuro Ophthalmol 2014;34(1):95–104.
21. Jang SH, Kim SH, Seo YS. Injury of the optic radiation in patients with mild TBI: A DTT study. Transl Neurosci 2020;11(1):335–40.
22. Kolbe S, Bajraszewski C, Chapman C, et al. Diffusion tensor imaging of the optic radiations after optic neuritis. Hum Brain Mapp 2012;33(9):2047–61.
23. Kolbe SC, Marriott M, van der Walt A, et al. Diffusion Tensor Imaging Correlates of Visual Impairment in Multiple Sclerosis and Chronic Optic Neuritis. Invest Ophthalmol Vis Sci 2012;53:825–32.
24. DeYoe EA, Carman GJ, Bandettini P, et al. Mapping striate and extrastriate visual areas in human cerebral cortex. Proc Natl Acad Sci U S A 1996;93(6): 2382–6.

25. Wu X, Kirov II, Gonen O, et al. MR Imaging applications in mild traumatic brain injury: an imaging update. Radiology 2016;279(3):693–707.

26. Kubas B, Lebkowski W, Lebkowski U, et al. Proton MR spectroscopy in mild traumatic brain injury. Pol J Radiol 2010;75(4):7–10.

27. Mao Y, Zhuang Z, Chen Y, et al. Imaging of glutamate in acute traumatic brain injury using chemical exchange saturation transfer. Quant Imaging Med Surg 2019;9(10):1652–63.

28. Lin CM, Tseng YC, Hsu HL, et al. Arterial spin labeling perfusion study in the patients with subacute mild traumatic brain injury. PLoS One 2016;11(2): e0149109.

29. Waitzman DM, Oliver DL. "Midbrain." Encyclopedia of the Human Brain, Ramachandran V.S. editor, Academic Press, Amsterdam, 2002, pp. 43–68.

Cerebrovascular Reactivity and Concussion

Erin T. Wong, MD[a,b], Anish Kapadia, MD[a,b], Venkatagiri Krishnamurthy, PhD[c,d,e], David J. Mikulis, MD[a,f,*]

KEYWORDS

• Cerebrovascular reactivity • Cerebral blood flow • Concussion • Traumatic brain injury

KEY POINTS

• Cerebrovascular reactivity (CVR) reflects the change in cerebral blood flow in response to a vaso-dilatory stimulus and therefore enables assessment of the health of the cerebral vasculature.
• Recent advances in the quantitative delivery of CO_2 stimuli with computer-controlled sequential gas delivery have enabled mapping of speed of response and magnitude of response CVR metrics.
• The exaggerated CVR response in the acute and subacute phases of concussion may relate to neu-rogliovascular uncoupling due to microstructural injury.
• The faster speed of response and greater magnitude of response in concussion have not been demonstrated in other diseases, which typically show the opposite effects.
• Alterations in CVR can persist into the chronic phase of concussion in symptomatic patients which raises the possibility of an association between ongoing blood flow dysregulation and impaired recovery.

INTRODUCTION TO CEREBROVASCULAR REACTIVITY
Overview of Cerebrovascular Physiology

Cerebral blood flow (CBF) is tightly regulated involving the interplay of numerous cellular elements, including endothelial cells, smooth muscle cells, and glial cells, which form the neurogliovascular unit (NGVU). There are also contributions from microglia and pericytes, although the contribution from pericytes is controversial. Importantly, the interplay between these cellular elements is not fully understood, but the final effector mechanism of the NGVU is smooth muscle tone influenced by intracellular hydrogen ion concentration.[1,2] Decreased perivascular pH also causes the relaxation of arteriolar smooth muscle through the reduction of intracellular calcium[3] (Fig. 1). As smooth muscle tone of the arteries and arterioles controls the diameter of blood vessels, this changes resistance to blood flow. In addition, each of the cellular elements can influence smooth muscle tone. Nitric oxide (NO) is a smooth muscle relaxant released during signaling affecting vascular homeostasis.[4] Endothelial cells constantly release NO modulated by a variety of stimuli. Glial cells can modulate smooth muscle tone based on the levels of neural activity and changes in dissolved substances, including oxygen and carbon dioxide (CO_2), among others. It is currently thought that smooth muscle cells can react to changes in blood pressure via a stretch reflex mechanism that does not necessarily involve the other components of the NGVU. However, the underlying physiology of

[a] Department of Medical Imaging, University of Toronto, Toronto, Ontario, Canada; [b] Department of Medical Imaging, Sunnybrook Health Sciences Centre, 2075 Bayview Avenue, Toronto, Ontario M4N 3M5, Canada; [c] Department of Medicine, Division of Geriatrics and Gerontology, Emory University, Atlanta, GA, USA; [d] Center for Visual and Neurocognitive Rehabilitation, Atlanta Veterans Affairs Medical Center (VAMC), 1670 Clairmont Road, Suite # 12C 141, Decatur, GA 30033, USA; [e] Department of Neurology, Emory University, Atlanta, GA, USA; [f] Department of Medical Imaging, University Health Network, Toronto Western Hospital, 399 Bathurst Street, Toronto, Ontario M5T 2S8, Canada
* Corresponding author. Department of Medical Imaging, Toronto Western Hospital, 399 Bathurst Street, Toronto, Ontario M5T 2S8, Canada.
E-mail address: david.mikulis@uhn.ca

Neuroimag Clin N Am 33 (2023) 335–342
https://doi.org/10.1016/j.nic.2023.01.008

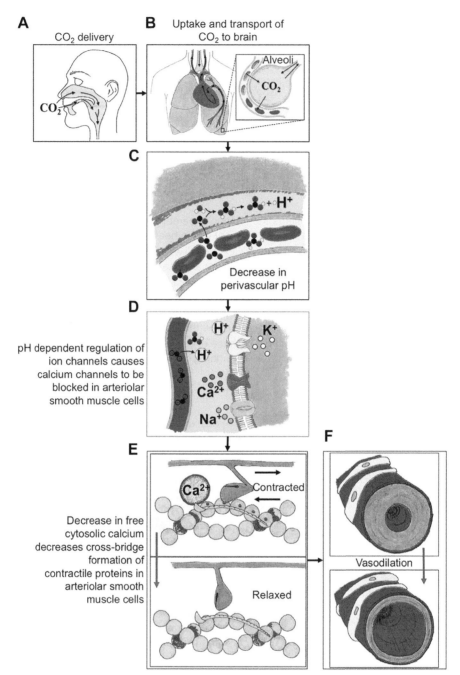

Fig. 1. Diagram demonstrating the physiological mechanism of carbon dioxide (CO_2) stimulus-related cerebrovascular reactivity (CVR). (*A*) Delivery of CO_2 to the participants' nasal and oral cavity. (*B*) Inspiration of CO_2 and mixing in the alveoli, with subsequent gas exchange and transport to the brain via the blood. (*C*) CO_2 exchange into the perivascular space from the blood decreasing perivascular pH. (*D*) Lowering pH results in the inhibition of calcium channels in arteriolar smooth muscle cells. (*E*) The resultant reduction in calcium concentration leads to the relaxation of arteriolar smooth muscle cells. (*F*) This results in local vasodilation and increased cerebral blood flow seen on MR imaging. Ca2+, calcium; H+, proton; K+, potassium; and Na+, sodium. (*From* Krishnamurthy V, Sprick JD, Krishnamurthy LC, et al. The Utility of Cerebrovascular Reactivity MRI in Brain Rehabilitation: A Mechanistic Perspective. Front Physiol. 2021;12:642850. Published 2021 Mar 17.)

this mechanism is not fully understood, and a complete description of NGVU function is beyond the scope of this overview.

Cerebrovascular reactivity (CVR) is defined as the change in CBF in response to a vasodilatory stimulus. It indicates the capacity of the cerebral blood vessels to dilate or constrict in response to various stimuli, thereby providing an assessment of the impact of both vascular and extravascular diseases on CBF regulation.[2] Measuring CVR ideally depends on the ability to selectively influence the vascular smooth muscle component of the NGVU without significantly changing neuronal activity. During stimulation, it is assumed that blood pressure and neuronal activity remain stable during the measurement. Hypotension can also be used as a vasoactive stimulus to measure CVR, although this is not easy to implement safely, especially in patients with cardiovascular or cerebrovascular disease.

Methods to measure cerebrovascular reactivity
A variety of methods have been used to measure CVR including variations in the delivery of vasoactive stimuli and measurement of changes in CBF. The most common methods for changing intracellular pH include the administration of acetazolamide and changing the arterial partial pressure of CO_2 ($PaCO_2$). Acetazolamide blocks carbonic anhydrase leading to an inability to convert bicarbonate and hydrogen ion to CO_2 and water for transfer into the blood, thereby decreasing intracellular pH that then influences the calcium concentration and smooth muscle contractility. Increasing $PaCO_2$ can be achieved by breath holding or increasing levels of inspired CO_2.

Blood oxygen-level-dependent (BOLD) MR imaging, arterial spin-labeling (ASL) MR imaging, phase-contrast (PC) MR imaging, and CT/single photon emission computed tomography (SPECT)/PET perfusion imaging are among the imaging methods used to map blood flow.[5] PC MR imaging and transcranial Doppler ultrasound have been used to measure blood velocity in large intracranial vessels, but they cannot map CVR at the whole-brain tissue level.

Given the heterogeneity of the stimuli and the methods of blood flow measurement, it is important to recognize the value of quantitation. To date, there is only one method available for delivering quantitative CO_2 stimuli while maintaining isoxia, that is, computer-controlled sequential gas delivery (SGD) via a sealed face mask. This method is unique in having end-tidal PCO_2 ($PETCO_2$) targets validated against arterial blood gas sampling.[6] In terms of blood flow measurement at the tissue level, PET is the gold standard, but it is not readily available as it requires a cyclotron to generate the needed radioactive tracers. Other available methods, including Computed Tomography (CT) or MR imaging bolus contrast perfusion imaging and ASL, tend to lose accuracy as the extent of vascular disease increases. Hopefully, future advances in ASL may soon meet these needs. Currently, BOLD imaging, identical to that used for measuring flow changes during functional MR imaging (fMR imaging) paradigms, is considered a reasonable surrogate for measuring changes in blood flow.

CVR mapping therefore remains semiquantitative at best, even when applying well-controlled stimuli. In spite of this, a significant advance provided by the SGD method is that it can deliver one breath "step" increases in $PETCO_2$ that enable measurement of a speed of response metric (modeled as an exponential rise in blood flow), in addition to the traditional magnitude of response metric thus yielding two measures of vascular performance.[5] The CO_2 stimulus protocol using SGD control for arterial blood gasses during BOLD MR imaging described by Shafi and colleagues in the setting of acute concussion involves: (1) 120 second of normocapnia at the subject's resting baseline $PETCO_2$, (2) 120 seconds of hypercapnia with a "step" increase 10 mm Hg above resting typically achieved in one breath, (3) 120 seconds of normocapnia at baseline, (4) 60 seconds of hypocapnia 5 mm Hg or greater below resting, (5) 240 second duration "ramp" increase to 15 mm Hg above baseline, and (6) 120 seconds of normocapnia at baseline $PETCO_2$ (Fig. 2). CVR maps can then be generated for the magnitude from the ramp stimulus and speed of response from the step stimulus (Fig. 3).

CVR has many potential clinical applications. These are divided into applications examining steno-occlusive diseases of large vessels and diseases that affect the parenchymal arteries of the brain. Changes in small vessel performance have been seen in healthy aging, cerebral small vessel disease related to vascular risk factors, sickle cell disease, parenchymal vascular malformations, Alzheimer's dementia, mitochondrial disorders, concussion, migraine, obstructive sleep apnea, and COVID-19 brain fog.

CONCUSSION
Definition and Diagnostic Criteria

Concussion, an uncomplicated form of mild traumatic brain injury (mTBI), is a major cause of disability among adults and children and makes up 80% to 90% of all TBI.[7] Many definitions of concussion based on clinical criteria have been

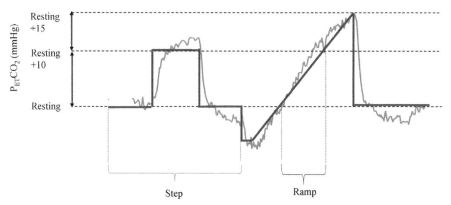

Fig. 2. Schematic of the targeted changes (*red line*) in end-tidal partial pressure of CO_2 (PETCO$_2$). The actual blood oxygen-level-dependent signal observed in a healthy subject (*blue line*). Note that 10 mm Hg changes in PETCO$_2$ are typically achieved in one breath followed by an exponential rise in the BOLD signal tissue response. (*From* Shafi R, Poublanc J, Venkatraghavan L, et al. A Promising Subject-Level Classification Model for Acute Concussion Based on Cerebrovascular Reactivity Metrics. J Neurotrauma. 2021;38(8):1036-1047.)

described. These predominantly originate from the sports literature, but most share common features and can be extrapolated to other mechanisms of injury. The most common definition based on the Concussion in Sport Group consensus statement describes a direct or indirect biomechanical force to the brain with physiological disruption of brain function manifesting in various clinical signs and symptoms that include, but are not limited to, confusion, disorientation, slowed thinking, and transient loss of consciousness.[8] Neurological impairment should be clearly related to the injury and not attributable to other causes (eg, alcohol, illicit drugs, medications, other injuries, comorbidities).[7] A drawback of the various clinical definitions of concussion has been the resultant lack

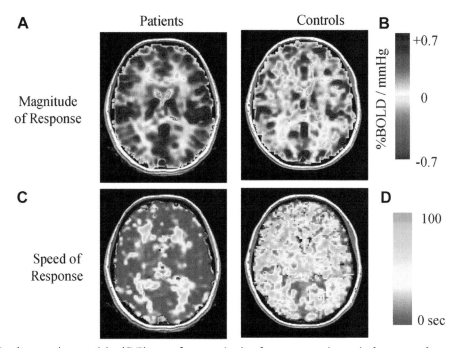

Fig. 3. Cerebrovascular reactivity (CVR) maps for magnitude of response and speed of response for a concussed patient (*A, C*) and a healthy control (*B, D*). The patient's scan demonstrates a higher CVR magnitude (*A* versus *B*) and an increased speed of response (*C* versus *D*) compared with the control. (*From* Shafi R, Poublanc J, Venkatraghavan L, et al. A Promising Subject-Level Classification Model for Acute Concussion Based on Cerebrovascular Reactivity Metrics. J Neurotrauma. 2021;38(8):1036-1047.)

of a gold standard to assess them diagnostically. Conventional neuroimaging studies (i.e., CT, MR imaging) of concussed patients are normal, revealing no macro-structural abnormality.[7,9] These techniques cannot detect the microstructural injuries that result in the acute neurological impairment present in concussed individuals. Therefore, the primary role of MR imaging has been in the chronic setting of head injury as it can provide evidence of brain trauma including contusions, cerebral atrophy, or parenchymal microhemorrhages that, according to the Panwar classification, indicate a greater injury severity than concussion alone.

Pathophysiology

Concussion occurs due to acceleration or deceleration of the head with resultant shear strain on the brain parenchyma.[10–12] These forces cause temporary disruption of axonal membranes with efflux of intracellular potassium and subsequent diffuse neuronal depolarization.[10] Excitatory neurotransmitters, namely glutamate, are released into the extracellular space that stimulates further potassium efflux and depolarization. Glutamate release also leads to the intraneuronal accumulation of sodium and calcium that can cause cell damage and mitochondrial dysfunction.[10] Reduced CBF has been reported changes in ion flux and neurotransmitter release.[13] The proposed mechanisms for decreased CBF include disruption of the NGVU, autoregulation, and autonomic regulation.[13] These effects result in a mismatch between excitatory phenomena and energy supply (from reduced glucose delivery).[12] The degree to which this results in permanent neuronal injury remains uncertain.

Clinical Signs and Symptoms

There are many signs and symptoms of concussion which can be divided into acute, subacute, and chronic phases. Acute clinical symptoms generally have a rapid onset but can sometimes begin minutes or hours after the inciting event.[8] Immediate structural injury, metabolic changes, neuroinflammation, and blood flow dysregulation can lead to the loss of consciousness, amnesia, confusion, disorientation, headache, and unsteadiness, among many other signs and symptoms.[12,14] Although most individuals spontaneously recover within 7 to 10 days (often within 3 days), long-term problems can persist.[13,15] Subacute and chronic signs/symptoms may fall into the following categories: affective/emotional (eg, anxiety, depression, irritability), cognitive (eg, confusion, difficulty concentrating, difficulty remembering, disorientation), sleep (eg,

drowsiness, decreased/increased sleep), and somatic/physical (eg, blurred vision, dizziness, fatigue, headache, nausea, light/noise sensitivity).[7] The subacute phase involves the repair of damaged neuronal networks, resolution of inflammation, and restoration of blood flow control. The vast majority (>95%) of individuals with concussion recover within the 3-month subacute period.[16] The chronic phase or persistent post-concussion syndrome (PCS) occurs when symptoms continue for over 3 months beyond the inciting brain injury.[17] Risk factors for the development of PCS include prior psychiatric disorder, older age, children and adolescents, female sex, and pre-injury health system usage.[18] The most important predictor may simply be the number of initial symptoms.[19] Management of PCS is primarily focused on symptom relief with non-pharmacological and pharmacologic interventions.[17] In many patients with PCS, symptoms persist for years and may not fully resolve. A higher number of initial symptoms is associated with a lower rate of recovery.[19]

Biomarkers and Diagnostic Tests

Advanced neuroimaging (eg, PET, SPECT, fMRI imaging, CVR), biochemical markers, and genetic testing are potential adjuncts to clinical evaluation that may allow for a more objective definition of concussion in the future.[8] Functional and metabolic imaging modalities may reveal abnormalities that reflect the microscopic or molecular pathologic changes that occur in mTBI.[20] PET imaging can detect abnormal glucose metabolism in mTBI which increases in the acute phase and decreases in the chronic phase.[20] SPECT has been studied in the diagnosis of TBI and may show focal areas of hypoperfusion not detectable on conventional CT or MR imaging.[21] Although the negative predictive value of SPECT is nearly 100%, the positive predictive value shortly after trauma was only 59% in one study.[22] Both PET and SPECT have relatively low spatial resolution in addition to potential issues with the standardization of image interpretation, data acquisition, and quantitative analysis, which may impact diagnostic reliability. Moreover, SPECT scans can demonstrate significant regional variability in radiotracer uptake even in normal adult subjects.[23] fMR imaging techniques in mTBI can detect changes in regional vascular activity and oxygen consumption in the resting state and during task-based paradigms.[20] The routine clinical use of fMR imaging is limited by cost, motion sensitivity, and MR imaging contraindications (eg, metal implants or foreign bodies). The emerging role of CVR in concussion will be further discussed in the following sections.

Multiple potential diagnostic fluid and genetic biomarkers have been studied but are not currently routinely used in clinical practice. A recent study of collegiate athletes found elevated blood levels of glial fibrillary acidic protein, ubiquitin C-terminal hydrolase-L1, and tau in athletes with concussion compared with preseason baseline levels and control athletes.[24] Several other blood biomarkers have also been found to be significantly altered in the setting of sport-related concussion (eg, α-amino-3-hydroxy-5-methyl-4-isoxazolepropionic acid receptor peptide, S100 calcium binding protein B (s100B), marinobufagenin, plasma soluble cellular prion protein, neuron-specific enolase, and calpain-derived αII-spectrin N-terminal fragment).[24] Salivary cortisol has not been shown to significantly differ between concussed athletes and controls.[25] One study of CSF biomarkers found increased neurofilament light protein and reduced amyloid β in professional ice hockey players with repeated mTBI and PCS, potentially related to axonal white matter injury and amyloid deposition.[26] Lastly, there is also emerging evidence that genetic variation may modulate immune and inflammatory pathways, hypothalamic-adrenal-pituitary axis function, symptom severity, and recovery times.[27,28]

CEREBROVASCULAR REACTIVITY AND CONCUSSION

Concussion remains a clinical diagnosis largely dependent on the subjective reporting of symptoms from the patient. A reliable objective biomarker is lacking, especially since conventional clinical imaging studies are normal. Advanced imaging has been able to identify microstructural changes and functional alterations using group comparisons between concussed and heathy control groups. A concussion diagnosis at the individual subject level is not yet possible. These techniques have promoted an understanding of the sequelae of injury but are insufficient for diagnostic use or prognostication. As described above, CVR is a reflection of the ability of the vasculature to respond to blood flow demand and can serve as a marker of cerebrovascular reserve. Importantly, impaired CVR in the setting of concussion has been recognized since the early 2000s.[29,30] Recent studies have begun to identify CVR as a potentially useful objective marker to diagnose concussion.[31,32]

Tegeler and colleagues noted impaired CVR in the setting of mTBI even after normal neurocognitive function was restored.[29] Using transcranial Doppler ultrasound, Len and colleagues[30] demonstrated impaired CVR in patients with mTBI during breath hold challenges or hyperventilation. More recently, CVR mapping using precise control of CO_2 stimuli via an SGD circuit during BOLD MR imaging has shown greater accuracy and reproducibility.[33] Using this technique, a wider range in the magnitude of CVR responses was observed (both higher and lower in the same individual compared with controls) in the subacute to chronic phase of injury in those individuals suffering from PCS.[33] In fact, CVR metrics derived using this technique have been shown to have a very high degree of sensitivity and specificity during the subacute phase of concussion (0.867 and 0.778, respectively), exceeding the diagnostic utility of any other test in the context of concussion at that time.[31] This exaggerated response indicates disruption of blood flow control with findings replicated in different cohorts of concussion patients.[31,32]

Within the first week of concussion, there is an increase in CVR globally and more specifically involving the default mode network with associated changes in functional connectivity.[34] Increased amplitude and faster CVR responses have been observed within the first week of concussion.[5] Interestingly, CVR changes in this study were most apparent in the cerebral white matter with ROC (receiver operating characterisitc curve) area under the curve values of 0.94 and 0.90 in males and females, respectively.[5] The reason for this remains unclear. However, it is known that microstructural disruption of white matter on diffusion tensor imaging is present following concussion.[35] Hypothetically, autonomic fibers that project to the vasculature in the cerebral cortex from brainstem nuclei including the raphe nucleus and locus coeruleus could be vulnerable to concussive forces, resulting in flow dysregulation. Alternatively, concussive injury to glial cell processes with terminations on vascular structures could confer a diminished ability of the glia to influence blood flow control.

The utility of CVR in the diagnosis of concussion has been demonstrated primarily in the acute and subacute setting. Evidence for alteration of CVR in the chronic stage is more limited, although many patients with symptoms up to 993 days in the Mutch study[33] demonstrated evidence of blood flow dysregulation. This suggests that changes in CVR that persist into the chronic stage of concussive injury could impact the ability to fully recover. It has been proposed that the exaggerated response is the result of injury to the NGVU.[32] Specifically, injury to the glial cell population with proliferation and activation of microglia by the concussive event could result in abnormal responses to vasoactive stimuli. Downstream repercussions include altered oxygen delivery, either oversupply or undersupply, with the potential to cause oxidative damage via a free radical mechanism perpetuating neuroinflammation and/or secondary injury. The exaggerated CVR response also helps to explain some of the symptomatology including the regional headaches and migraine-type symptoms.

Future Directions

Advances in CVR mapping, particularly the ability to provide an accurate but rapidly changing flow stimulus, have enabled mapping of speed and magnitude of response metrics. These metrics have revealed a remarkable pattern of dysregulated blood flow control in individuals with acute concussion, who demonstrate faster speed and larger magnitude of responses unseen in other diseases that typically *slow* the speed and reduce the magnitude of response. Furthermore, dysregulated blood flow was present in those individuals who had persistent symptoms. This raises the possibility that persistent blood flow dysregulation could have a profound effect on recovery and may even be responsible for secondary injury through neurovascular uncoupling. Future research is warranted to examine these potential links. Continued CVR development could prove valuable for improving diagnosis, prognostication, and even assessment of treatment efficacy following concussion.

CLINICS CARE POINTS

- Recent work suggests that concussion is a subset of mTBI that is associated with an absence of abnormalities on conventional clinical inaging inlcuding CT and MRI.
- New evidence indicates that an unusual form of cerebral blood flow dysrequlation is present in individuals wirth acute concussion consisting of exagerated blood flow responses to vasoactive stimuli.

DISCLOSURE

This work was financially supported by the Holt-Hornsby and Andreae Vascular Dementia Research Unit in the Joint Department of Medical Imaging at the Toronto Western Hospital and the University Health Network.

REFERENCES

1. Duffin J, Mikulis DJ, Fisher JA. Control of cerebral blood flow by blood gases. Front Physiol 2021;12. Available at: https://www.frontiersin.org/articles/10.3389/fphys.2021.640075. Accessed July 19, 2022.

2. Sleight E, Stringer MS, Marshall I, et al. Cerebrovascular reactivity measurement using magnetic resonance imaging: a systematic review. Front Physiol 2021;12:643468.

3. Krishnamurthy V, Sprick JD, Krishnamurthy LC, et al. The utility of cerebrovascular reactivity MRI in brain rehabilitation: a mechanistic perspective. Front Physiol 2021;12:642850.

4. Ignarro LJ. Nitric oxide as a unique signaling molecule in the vascular system: a historical overview. J Physiol Pharmacol 2002;53(4 Pt 1):503–14.

5. Shafi R, Poublanc J, Venkatraghavan L, et al. a promising subject-level classification model for acute concussion based on cerebrovascular reactivity metrics. J Neurotrauma 2021;38(8):1036–47.

6. Ito S, Mardimae A, Han J, et al. Non-invasive prospective targeting of arterial P in subjects at rest. J Physiol 2008;586(15):3675–82.

7. Scorza KA, Raleigh MF, O'Connor FG. Current concepts in concussion: evaluation and management. Am Fam Physician 2012;85(2):123–32.

8. McCrory P, Feddermann-Demont N, Dvořák J, et al. What is the definition of sports-related concussion: a systematic review. Br J Sports Med 2017;51(11):877–87.

9. Panwar J, Hsu CCT, Tator CH, et al. Magnetic resonance imaging criteria for post-concussion syndrome: a study of 127 post-concussion syndrome patients. J Neurotrauma 2020;37(10):1190–6.

10. Romeu-Mejia R, Giza CC, Goldman JT. Concussion pathophysiology and injury biomechanics. Curr Rev Musculoskelet Med 2019;12(2):105–16.

11. Shaw NA. The neurophysiology of concussion. Prog Neurobiol 2002;67(4):281–344.

12. Stillman A, Alexander M, Mannix R, et al. Concussion: evaluation and management. Cleve Clin J Med 2017;84(8):623–30.

13. Wang Y, Nelson LD, LaRoche AA, et al. Cerebral blood flow alterations in acute sport-related concussion. J Neurotrauma 2016;33(13):1227–36.

14. Patterson ZR, Holahan MR. Understanding the neuroinflammatory response following concussion to develop treatment strategies. Front Cell Neurosci 2012;6:58.

15. Leddy JJ, Sandhu H, Sodhi V, et al. Rehabilitation of concussion and post-concussion syndrome. Sports Health 2012;4(2):147–54.

16. Kara S, Crosswell H, Forch K, et al. Less than half of patients recover within 2 weeks of injury after a sports-related mild traumatic brain injury: a 2-year prospective study. Clin J Sport Med 2020;30(2):96–101.

17. Polinder S, Cnossen MC, Real RGL, et al. A multidimensional approach to post-concussion symptoms in mild traumatic brain injury. Front Neurol 2018;9:1113.

18. Langer LK, Alavinia SM, Lawrence DW, et al. Prediction of risk of prolonged post-concussion symptoms: derivation and validation of the TRICORDRR (Toronto Rehabilitation Institute Concussion Outcome Determination and Rehab Recommendations) score. PLoS Med 2021;18(7):e1003652.

19. Tator CH, Davis HS, Dufort PA, et al. Postconcussion syndrome: demographics and predictors in 221 patients. J Neurosurg 2016;125(5):1206–16.

20. Shin SS, Bales JW, Edward Dixon C, et al. Structural imaging of mild traumatic brain injury may not be enough: overview of functional and metabolic imaging of mild traumatic brain injury. Brain Imaging Behav 2017; 11(2):591–610.

21. Raji CA, Tarzwell R, Pavel D, et al. Clinical utility of SPECT neuroimaging in the diagnosis and treatment of traumatic brain injury: a systematic review. PLoS One 2014;9(3):e91088.

22. Jacobs A, Put E, Ingels M, et al. Prospective evaluation of technetium-99m-HMPAO SPECT in mild and moderate traumatic brain injury. J Nucl Med 1994; 35(6):942–7.

23. Tanaka F, Vines D, Tsuchida T, et al. Normal patterns on 99mTc-ECD brain SPECT scans in adults. J Nucl Med 2000;41(9):1456–64.

24. McCrea M, Broglio SP, McAllister TW, et al. Association of blood biomarkers with acute sport-related concussion in collegiate athletes: findings from the NCAA and department of defense CARE consortium. JAMA Netw Open 2020;3(1):e1919771.

25. Hutchison MG, Mainwaring L, Senthinathan A, et al. Psychological and physiological markers of stress in concussed athletes across recovery milestones. J Head Trauma Rehabil 2017;32(3):E38–48.

26. Shahim P, Tegner Y, Gustafsson B, et al. Neurochemical aftermath of repetitive mild traumatic brain injury. JAMA Neurol 2016;73(11):1308–15.

27. McCrea M, Meier T, Huber D, et al. Role of advanced neuroimaging, fluid biomarkers and genetic testing in the assessment of sport-related concussion: a systematic review. Br J Sports Med 2017;51(12): 919–29.

28. Miller MR, Robinson M, Fischer L, et al. Putative Concussion Biomarkers Identified in Adolescent Male Athletes Using Targeted Plasma Proteomics. Front Neurol 2021;12. Available at: https://www.frontiersin.org/articles/10.3389/fneur.2021.787480. Accessed July 19, 2022.

29. Abstracts of the European Society of Neurosonology and Cerebral Hemodynamics. Wetzlar, Germany, May 9-11, 2004. Cerebrovasc Dis Basel Switz 2004;17(Suppl 4):1–38.

30. Len TK, Neary JP, Asmundson GJG, et al. Cerebrovascular reactivity impairment after sport-induced concussion. Med Sci Sports Exerc 2011;43(12): 2241–8.

31. Mutch WAC, Ellis MJ, Ryner LN, et al. Patient-specific alterations in CO_2 cerebrovascular responsiveness in acute and sub-acute sports-related concussion. Front Neurol 2018;9:23.

32. Wang R, Poublanc J, Crawley AP, et al. Cerebrovascular reactivity changes in acute concussion: a controlled cohort study. Quant Imaging Med Surg 2021;11(11):4530–42.

33. Mutch WAC, Ellis MJ, Ryner LN, et al. Brain magnetic resonance imaging CO_2 stress testing in adolescent postconcussion syndrome. J Neurosurg 2016; 125(3):648–60.

34. Militana AR, Donahue MJ, Sills AK, et al. Alterations in default-mode network connectivity may be influenced by cerebrovascular changes within one week of sports related concussion in college varsity athletes: a pilot study. Brain Imaging Behav 2016; 10(2):559–68.

35. Wilde EA, Goodrich-Hunsaker NJ, Ware AL, et al. Diffusion tensor imaging indicators of white matter injury are correlated with a multimodal electroencephalography-based biomarker in slow recovering, concussed collegiate athletes. J Neurotrauma 2020;37(19):2093–101.

The Current State of Susceptibility-Weighted Imaging and Quantitative Susceptibility Mapping in Head Trauma

Charlie Chia-Tsong Hsu, MBBS, FRANZCR[a,b,*], Sean K. Sethi, MS[c],
E. Mark Haacke, PhD[c,d]

KEYWORDS

- Traumatic brain injury (TBI) • Concussion • Post-concussion syndrome (PCS)
- Susceptibility-weighted imaging (SWI) • Quantitative susceptibility mapping (QSM)
- Artificial intelligence (AI)

KEY POINTS

- Review the physics principles of susceptibility-weighted imaging (SWI) and the evolution of blood degradation products.
- SWI is a sensitive MR imaging sequence for the detection of microbleeds, which is a biomarker of traumatic brain injury (TBI). Number and volume of microbleeds in TBI correlate with clinical outcome and morbidity.
- Concussion and post-concussion syndrome have no or weak association with microbleeds. The role of SWI in this circumstance may serve to exclude TBI and to facilitate a return to sport and activity.
- Understand the steps in quantitative susceptibility mapping (QSM) and the scalar quantity of susceptibility (ppm) of basic substances.
- Review the emerging applications of QSM and artificial intelligence in the detection and quantification of microbleeds.

INTRODUCTION

Neuroimaging performed in the setting of head injuries assists clinicians in classifying the severity of injury, identifying structural brain lesions for the treatment of patients' traumatic brain injury (TBI), and preventing secondary injury. For acute head injury, the appropriate initial examination is a non-contrast computed tomography (CT) head scan, which serves to exclude intra-axial or extra-axial hemorrhage, brain contusion, and brain herniation all of which may necessitate urgent neurosurgical intervention. MR imaging with conventional and advanced techniques provides a more in-depth assessment of the severity of TBI than CT and provides prognostic information for clinicians. In this article, we discuss the basic principles of susceptibility-weighted imaging (SWI) and quantitative susceptibility mapping (QSM), as well as their application to TBI.

[a] Division of Neuroradiology, Department of Medical Imaging, Gold Coast University Hospital, Australia;
[b] Division of Neuroradiology, Lumus Imaging, Varsity Lakes Day Hospital, Gold Coast, Australia;
[c] Department of Radiology, Wayne State University School of Medicine; [d] Department of Neurology, Wayne State University School of Medicine
* Corresponding author. Division of Neuroradiology, Varsity Lakes Day Hospital, Gold Coast, Australia.
E-mail addresses: charlie.ct.hsu@gmail.com; charlie.hsu@health.qld.gov.au

Neuroimag Clin N Am 33 (2023) 343–356
https://doi.org/10.1016/j.nic.2023.01.009
1052-5149/23/© 2023 Elsevier Inc. All rights reserved.

The Pathophysiology and Biomechanics of Traumatic Brain Injury

Understanding the biomechanics of TBI has an important bearing on the pattern of injury seen in MR imaging. The brain is contained within a rigid skull vault surrounded by cerebrospinal fluid (CSF) that cushions the brain during mechanical motion. In the event of head trauma, the external forces generate pressure gradients on the brain either as direct impact or indirectly in the form of acceleration-deceleration. A complex combination of linear and rotational forces is transmitted through the noncompressible CSF onto the brain surface causing deformation of the elastic brain surface as well as the internal shift of brain substance.[1] Transmitted forces from the noncompressible CSF impact the brain's surface. The degree of brain deformability depends on the strength of the force, brain geometry, and anatomic variation of the rigidity of the brain's tissue. The brain's surface is not uniform having gyral ridges and sulcations.[2] The bases of the sulci are exposed to the highest force, the so-called water hammer effect.[2] The parallel orientation of the axons at the base of the sulci assists in dissipating the transmitted energy but the different rigidity interfaces between the cortical gray matter and white matter results in shearing axonal and vascular injuries.[2] The surface of the brain can also be driven against the noncompressible cranial vault, especially at the skull base leading to contusions.[1]

At the biochemical level, in the acute phase, TBI leads to a rapid neuronal depolarization characterized by the release of excitatory neurotransmitters such as glutamate and activation of N-methyl-D-aspartate receptors.[1,3] The net effect promotes the intracellular influx of calcium ions and the efflux of potassium. The increased intracellular calcium has a negative consequence of activation of calcium-dependent proteases, mitochondrial dysfunction, and release of oxygen free radicals contributing to cellular injury.[1,3] The opposing cellular mechanism to restore the transmembrane ion gradient is through the action of the Na/K ATPase pump. The restorative process requires active transport but leads to an increase in cellular glucose utilization and anaerobic metabolism with an adverse accumulation of lactate and local acidosis. A cellular neuroinflammatory cascade also occurs simultaneously triggered by the release of intracellular signaling molecules (such as cytokines and complements). The cellular response leads to the activation of microglia and proteases and the generation of free radicals in a positive feedback cycle.

The inflammatory response also leads to increased permeability of the blood-brain barrier with the influx of the hematopoietic immune cells including neutrophils, macrophages, and lymphocytes.[3] Depending on the severity of the TBI, the neuroinflammatory process gradually tapers off over several months to years. Chronic neurologic sequelae from posttraumatic neuro-inflammation and structural injuries could lead to long-term dysregulation of neurotransmitters and ionic transports, membrane depolarization, upregulation of β-amyloid precursor protein (β-APP), and accumulation of tau protein.[4,5] These processes could form the basis for neurodegenerative diseases such as chronic traumatic encephalopathy.

PRINCIPLES OF SUSCEPTIBILITY-WEIGHTED IMAGING

SWI is a three-dimensional (3D), high-resolution, flow-compensated gradient echo sequence. The conventional SWI image is created through a series of mathematical steps to enhance the T2* effect of microbleeds, veins, calcifications, and other sources of local susceptibility.[6–8] First, the original phase data are unwrapped and then high pass filtered to remove background field variations caused by air/tissue interfaces and other low spatial frequency field inhomogeneities. This phase image is then turned into a phase mask with the property that, for a right-handed system (right vs left-handed systems will be discussed later). The phase mask f(x) is set to unity for phase values (φ (x)) between 0 and π and equal to (φ (x) + π)/ π for phase values from -π to 0. This phase mask $f(x)$ is then applied to the original long echo (usually approximately 20 to 25 ms) magnitude image $S(TE_{long})$ multiple times (usually four times) to reduce the signal in regions where the phase is significantly different from zero:

$$SWI(TE_{long}) = f(x)^4 S(TE_{long}) \qquad (1)$$

Finally, to allow the connectivity of the structures of interest, particularly the veins, an additional image, a minimum intensity projection (mIP), is generated by projecting the minimum signal over multiple slices (usually over four slices).

Generating contrast with gradient echo imaging is determined by the tissue properties and imaging parameters. The signal magnitude of the final SWI image is a function of T1, T2*, geometry, orientation of the veins to the main magnetic field (B_o), and the difference in phase between the tissues imaged. The magnitude signal for 3D gradient echo imaging before applying the phase mask is given by

$$S(TE) = \rho_o \sin\theta \ (1 - E1)/(1 - E1\cos\theta)\exp(-TE/T2^*) \tag{2}$$

where ρ_o is the tissue spin density, θ is the flip angle, $E1 = \exp(-TR/T1)$, TR is the repetition time, TE is the echo time, T1 is the longitudinal relaxation time, and T2* is the transverse relaxation time for a specific tissue. It is prudent to note that although T2* and phase effects dominate when blood is present, there is still a T1 term present when the flip angle is greater than or close to the Ernst angle ($\theta_E = \mathrm{sqrt}(2\ TR/T1)$). Hence, the SWI signal is influenced by both T2* and T1 effects both of which can be observed and accentuated by adjusting the MR parameters.

Different materials interact differently when placed in a magnetic field and they can be broadly designated as diamagnetic, paramagnetic, or ferromagnetic. For a right-handed system and for veins parallel to the main field, diamagnetic materials have negative susceptibility (positive phase shift), whereas paramagnetic and ferromagnetic materials have positive susceptibility (negative phase shift).[6–8] However, for small vessels less than a voxel in size, such as medullary veins perpendicular to the main field, the veins will show the same sign as when they are parallel to the field.

SUSCEPTIBILITY-WEIGHTED IMAGING PHYSICS OF CEREBRAL HEMORRHAGE

In TBI, vascular injury leads to the release of red blood cells (RBC) which, in turn, leads to a stepwise transformation process of hemoglobin degradation. Iron (Fe) in the hemoglobin molecule exhibits a different degree of paramagnetic susceptibility signal based on the number of unpaired electrons in the molecule. The iron in oxyhemoglobin has no unpaired electrons and exhibits a weak diamagnetic property. On the contrary, the iron in deoxyhemoglobin (Fe^{2+}) has four unpaired electrons and demonstrates strong paramagnetic effects. Subsequently, deoxyhemoglobin undergoes oxidation to methemoglobin (Fe^{3+}) with five unpaired electrons further accentuating its paramagnetic property. Blood products may eventually become deposited in brain tissue (within macrophages or glial cells) as hemosiderin. Hemosiderin is an amorphous insoluble form of ferritin. Each iron atom in ferritin has 3 unpaired electrons and each ferritin molecule contains on the order of 2000 iron atoms. Both ferritin and hemosiderin are superparamagnetic and when exposed to an external magnetic field, spins from the electrons combine to produce a marked magnetic susceptibility effect.

In TBI, cerebral hemorrhage can manifest as linear or dot-like microbleeds due to shearing axonal and vascular injuries (Fig. 1) or in the form of a lobar hematoma from contusions or rupture of larger size vessels. Understanding the SWI physics principles can better aid in hemorrhage characterization. It is essential to understand that the appearance of microbleeds on SWI can be variable depending on their size and geometry and, therefore, on the imaging resolution and available signal-to-noise.

The sign of the phase for diamagnetic and paramagnetic substances is vendor-specific.[7] Scanners with a left-handed reference frame (Siemens) show diamagnetic calcium as negative and paramagnetic heme products as positive, whereas the opposite is true for a right-handed reference frame (GE/Philips). The above observation holds for small spherical structures or cylinders parallel to the main field with homogenous susceptibility. Phase images themselves have the potential to differentiate paramagnetic microbleeds from calcifications which is important in the clinical context of TBI (Fig. 2). However, diagnostically it requires an understanding of the shape of the dipole field. One means to recognize this dipole effect is to look for a halo at the equator of the sphere.[9] For a right-handed system, this halo will be bright if it is a bleed or dark if a calcification.[9] You need to view the halo on the outermost ring when there is no more aliasing of the phase to make this determination (Fig. 3).[9]

Lobar hematomas can have a variable appearance on SWI. It was recognized in an early retrospective study that hyperintense signal intensity of cerebral hematomas was associated with increased T1-weighted signal.[10] This is due to a phenomenon known as the SWI "T1 shine through" effect. High intrinsic T1-weighted signal occurs in late subacute hematomas due to a higher concentration of methemoglobin, especially at the core of the hematoma and the predominate T1-relaxivity effect seems as hyperintense on SWI (Fig. 4). Although methemoglobin is highly paramagnetic with five unpaired electrons, the T2* effect is greater when compartmentalized within the RBC as noted in the early subacute phase. In contrast, the late subacute phase of a hematoma, the lysis of the RBC leads to the mixing of extracellular methemoglobin with serum nulling/reducing the T2/T2* effect. An important note to make is that the progress of hemoglobin degradation is not homogeneous with hemosiderin deposition occurring at the periphery of the hematoma at a faster pace due to greater immune cellular (microglia and macrophage) accessibility. On SWI, this is represented by an earlier development of a hypointense

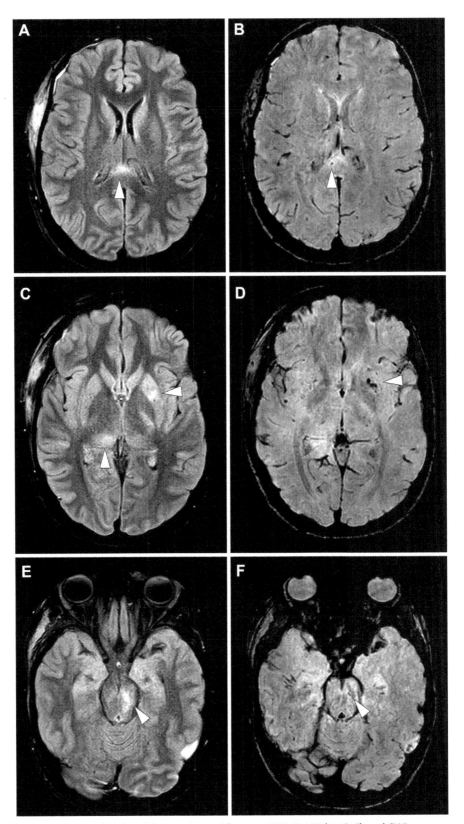

Fig. 1. Diffuse axonal injury (grade III) in a patient with severe TBI. FLAIR (*A*, *C*, *E*) and SWI sequences (*B*, *D*, *F*) reveal edema and microbleeds, respectively, with the edema being seen at the splenium of the corpus callosum, left putamen, pulvinar of the right thalamus and the left cerebral peduncle (*arrowheads*).

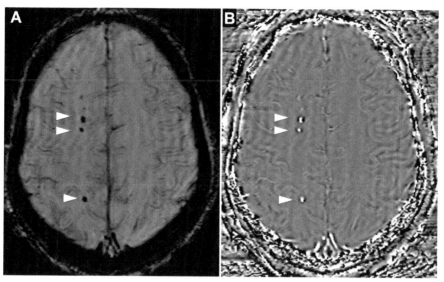

Fig. 2. Patient with TBI showing microbleeds in the right centrum semiovale. The SWI image (*A*) shows the signal loss in three of the larger lesions, whereas the phase image (*B*) shows a hyperintense (positive phase shift) center with a black outer halo indicating a paramagnetic effect. The MR imaging scan was obtained with a left-handed reference frame (Siemens 3.0 T Skyra, Erlangen, Germany).

rim that progresses slowly in a centripetal fashion as the hematoma involutes. Other processes that also contribute to the hypointense rim around a hematoma include the superparamagnetic susceptibility effect of hemosiderin, compartmentalization of hemosiderin within microglia or macrophages, and the difference in magnetic susceptibility between voxels containing hemosiderin and adjacent brain tissues surrounding the hematoma.[10,11]

MICROBLEEDS AND CLINICAL OUTCOME IN TRAUMATIC BRAIN INJURY

SWI is an ideal MR imaging sequence for imaging TBI due to its exquisite sensitivity for the detection of blood products (hemorrhage) and venous blood (a surrogate for deoxygenated hemoglobin concentration). SWI is superior to conventional T2* GRE sequence for traumatic hemorrhagic lesions, especially microbleeds.[12–14] More specifically, SWI has been shown to be more sensitive in the detection of traumatic hemorrhagic lesions than CT or conventional MR imaging sequences (CT scan detection rate 68%, conventional MR imaging 54%, and SWI in 86%).[15] When compared with the usual 2D T2*GRE sequence, 3D SWI has been shown to be more sensitive in detecting hemorrhagic lesions in patients with mild TBI.[16]

Microbleeds are imaging biomarkers of TBI. Total microbleed burden (number and volume) identified on SWI has clinical implications in patients after TBI. The number and volume of hemorrhagic lesions in adult patients with TBI correlate with

neurologic disability and impairment of global intelligence, memory, and attention.[17,18] Microbleeds may manifest as a punctate shape or seem linear and may suggest microvascular damage to the surrounding vascular tree after comparing MR imaging lesions with histologic staining for iron-laden macrophages in the perivascular spaces (Fig. 5).[19] Further, the presence of these trauma-induced microbleeds has been shown to be a predictor of disability, although it is not clear if this equates to axonal injury. SWI has increased sensitivity for hemorrhagic lesions in severe TBI compared with conventional MR imaging sequences (T1WI, T2WI, Fluid-attenuated inversion recovery [FLAIR], DWI, and T2* GRE), a finding that is significant for microbleeds less than 10 mm in diameter.[20] There is also a negative correlation between the number of hemorrhagic lesions detected on SWI and the Glasgow Coma Score (GCS) score, where the overall number of hemorrhagic lesions negatively correlates with the GCS score.[19]

Similarly, SWI for pediatric TBI patients may provide prognostic information regarding the duration of the coma as well as the long-term outcome. In a cohort study of 106 pediatric patients with varying TBI severity (mild, moderate, severe), the number and volume of hemorrhagic lesions on SWI correlated significantly with clinical outcome variables including GCS, surgical intervention, length of hospital stay and length of intubation and intellectual functioning in the initial stages post-injury (average 1 month).[21] Similar findings

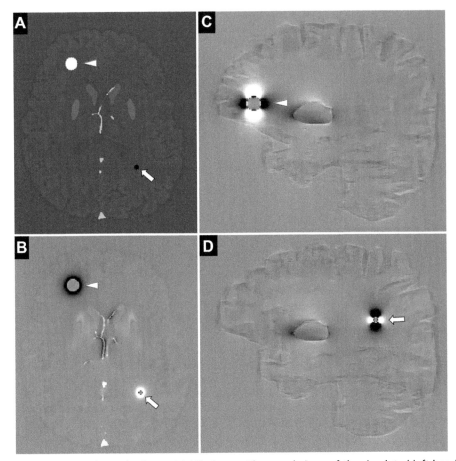

Fig. 3. Susceptibility map of a 3D brain model (A) along with several views of the simulated left-handed phase images (B–D) in the transverse (B) and sagittal (C, D) planes. A cerebral microbleed (*arrowhead*, radius = 5 mm, $\Delta\chi$ = 1 ppm) and a calcium deposit (*arrow*, radius 2 mm, $\Delta\chi$ = −3 ppm) were included in the white matter. The phase images were simulated with Bo = 3T and TE = 7.5 ms. Note the arrowhead and arrow in (C, D) point to the equatorial plane where the phase is shown in (B). Here the dark halo for the bleed a bright halo for the calcium indicates paramagnetic and diamagnetic, respectively. (*Courtesy of* S Buch, PhD, Detroit, MI.)

were also reported in a cohort of 40 pediatric patients with TBI demonstrating that a poorer clinical profile with a lower GCS score or prolonged coma has an increased number and volume of hemorrhagic lesions on SWI. On the contrary, children with normal outcomes or mild disability at 6 to 12 months had, on average, fewer and lower volumes of hemorrhagic lesions compared with moderate or severe TBI patients.[22] Microbleeds detected on SWI as a biomarker of mild TBI may need to be taken in the clinical context of the mechanism of injury. An interesting study of mild TBI in military service members showed that the occurrence of microbleeds as high as 28% in the acute and subacute stages following blunt-related mild TBI but no microbleeds were observed in the blast-related mild TBI.[23]

Concussion and mild TBI are prevalent and account for 75% of all reported cases of head injuries. Mild TBI is at the lower end of the spectrum of TBI and can show traumatic structural brain lesions such as microbleeds on SWI which has a positive correlation with clinical severity.[24] In a larger cohort study, the distribution of microbleeds in mild TBI patients showed more microbleeds on SWI than in the control group (87% vs 20%) and, interestingly, in the mild TBI group, there were more microbleeds in the cortex/subcortical region whilst the microbleeds were more centrally located in the control group. In addition, there was no statistical difference in the number of microbleeds in the cerebellum and brainstem.[18] This observation was confirmed in a retrospective study which showed microbleeds detected on SWI in mild TBI were located more frequently in white matter than in deep nuclei, where they tend to reside in controls.[25] In mild TBI, microbleed burden specifically in the frontal,

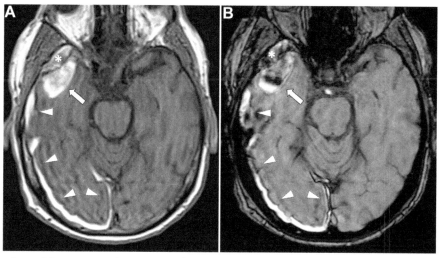

Fig. 4. A patient with severe TBI showing a multi-compartment right hemispheric subdural hematoma (*arrow-heads*), a right anterior temporal extradural hematoma (*asterisks*) and a right anterior temporal intraparenchy-mal hematoma (*arrow*). The T1-weighted image (*A*) shows the late subacute nature of the blood product appearing intrinsically hyperintense on the T1-weighted image. The T1-shine through is seen on the correspond-ing SWI image (*B*) with some area of the hemorrhage appearing hyperintense.

parietal and temporal lobes, was significantly greater in patients with clinical depression than in the non-depressive control group.[26]

On the contrary, in most cases of concussion, clinical symptoms resolved within 14 days. In a small subset of patients with concussion, 20%, do not fully recover and will have persistent symptoms beyond the initial one to 3 months which are designated to have post-concussion syndrome (PCS). In a study of 127 patients with PCS using T2* GRE sequence, posttraumatic lesions tended to be rare.[27] Only two patients with microbleeds and two patients with cortical encephalomalacia were found, which was not statistically significant compared with the controls.[27] However, the T2* GRE sequence may be less sensitive at depicting tiny microbleeds. In a separate study using SWI on a 3-T MR imaging platform, no microhemorrhages were detected as a result of a concussion or playing a season of ice hockey.[28] A small sample size study included 12 children who had experienced a single sports-related concussion, a

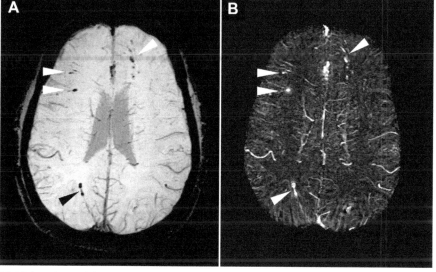

Fig. 5. mIP SWI (*A*) and QSM (*B*) images demonstrating punctate and linear morphology of microbleeds in bifrontal and right parietal region supportive of microvascular injury to the medullary veins.

qualitative review of the conventional and SWI MR imaging sequences did not reveal microbleeds or any other abnormalities.[29] A retrospective study of 151 pediatric sports-related concussions from a multidisciplinary tertiary hospital program also showed that the majority of neuroimaging studies (CT or MR imaging) are normal with only one case of intraparenchymal hemorrhage, a case of nonhemorrhagic contusion and few other nontraumatic incidental findings.[30] In both amateur boxers and professional athletes (National Football League players), there seems to be a weak association with microbleeds detected on SWI but not statistically significant. We must emphasize that the relative absence of hemorrhagic lesions in low-grade head injuries does not imply the absence of neural or axonal injury. The utility of conventional resolution SWI in low-grade head injuries may act as a screening tool to exclude more serious structural lesions. In the context of participation in contact sports, SWI MR imaging may have an impact on decision-making about a return to competition.

Subarachnoid Hemorrhage

SWI is a sensitive MR imaging sequence for the detection of acute traumatic subarachnoid hemorrhage (SAH). The paramagnetic property of the SAH is contrasted by the CSF signal intensity in the sulci, cisterns or within the ventricles, which has a susceptibility value near zero. Thin SAH seems as a gyriform paramagnetic signal base on the phase images (hyperintense on the left-handed MR imaging system and hypointense on the right-handed MR imaging system) but when the SAH is thicker it produces mixed hyper- and hypo-signal intensities due to phase aliasing (Fig. 6).[31] In the appropriate clinical context, SWI alone or in combination with FLAIR is more sensitive than CT for the depiction of subtle traumatic SAH.[32,33] Topographically, FLAIR was sensitive for the detection of frontoparietal, temporooccipital and Sylvian cistern SAH, whereas SWI was particularly sensitive for interhemispheric and intraventricular hemorrhage.[32]

Quantitative Susceptibility Mapping

QSM is an imaging technique that enables measurements of absolute concentrations of paramagnetic or diamagnetic substances in tissues based on changes in local susceptibility (Fig. 7). The QSM technique uses at least one echo for the detection of phase changes representative of susceptibility changes. In QSM, typically, several echoes are acquired with TEs ranging from 10 to 44 ms for 1.5 T and 5 to 25 ms for 3T with flow compensation in the readout direction. Several models have been developed to analyze QSM data.[6] In QSM, the unwanted background field contribution to the MR imaging phase image is removed by the appropriate filtering. One popular method for phase processing is the sophisticated harmonic artifact reduction for phase data (SHARP). Calculation of the total phase shift in a voxel depends on a complex interaction of structural geometry, composition, and orientation. A simplistic conceptualization would be to depict the susceptibility signals from paramagnetic or diamagnetic material within the image voxel as a magnetic dipole that interacts with the surrounding environment to create a local susceptibility field disturbance that extends beyond the voxel itself. Dipole fields originating from different voxels follow the superposition rule resulting in a convolution relationship between field and susceptibility that can be expressed as a multiplication of the Fourier transform of the source susceptibility and the Green's function in k-space. The final step in obtaining the QSM results requires solving the inverse problem to obtain the source distribution spatially. Unfortunately, solving the inverse problem is ill-posed because the Green's function has zeroes that must be regularized.

Several software QSM algorithms have been developed to address this issue from the simple threshold k-space approach to more complicated approaches such as MEDI and scSWIM.[34,35] Both SWI and QSM are output from the strategically acquired gradient echo (STAGE) protocol which uses either a single or multi-echo approach and became the first FDA-approved QSM technique (Fig. 8). QSM software computes the underlying susceptibility of each voxel as a scalar quantity. On QSM images, relative to water, a high signal represents paramagnetic susceptibility and a low signal represents diamagnetic susceptibility.

The susceptibility of water is −9.03 ppm at body temperature, whereas the susceptibility of air is roughly 0.35 ppm. The white matter in the brain appears to have a phase equal to roughly 0 ppm in QSM (with other tissues varying from a few dozen ppb to several 100ppb when iron is present) whereas the susceptibility at the air/tissue interfaces is dramatically higher being 9.4 ppm.[8,36] Example susceptibilities (in SI units) for different materials of interest within the brain are as follows: calcium (Ca2+ hydroxyapatite) (−14.83 ppm, which is equivalent to −5.8 ppm with respect to water. On the contrary, measurement of calcium susceptibility in human bone using QSM yields roughly −3 ppm with reference to water or surrounding tissues), the difference between fully deoxygenated and oxygenated blood (3.43 ppm), methemoglobin

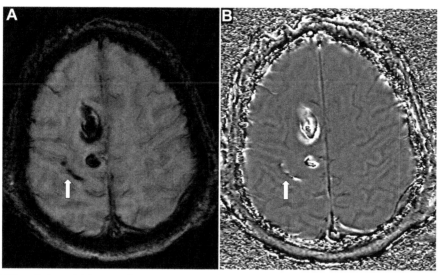

Fig. 6. SWI (*A*) and phase (*B*) images showing traumatic cerebral contusion in the right superior frontal gyrus and rather conspicuous sulcal SAH along the right central sulcus (*arrow*). Note the phase aliasing of the SAH in the phase image (*arrow*).

(3.72 ppm), ferritin core (2011 ppm fully loaded), hemosiderin (1578 ppm, based on the ratio of its molar susceptibility to that of ferritin).[8,36] The final susceptibility for brain tissue will depend on the concentration of these substances. For example, if the fraction of ferritin is only 0.001 then the susceptibility in the tissue will be just 2 ppm. To complicate matters further this also depends on the loading of iron in the ferritin so these numbers are only estimates.

with the controls.[38] The increased susceptibility signal in the cerebral venous structures may be due to venous stasis, enlarged or damaged veins, extravasated blood, or micro-thrombosis around the vessel wall. The segmented venous volume also encompasses some perivascular and deep white matter areas. This increase might be attributed to representing the damage in the perivascular regions associated with iron deposition or astroglial scarring.[38]

Applications of Quantitative Susceptibility Mapping in Traumatic Brain Injury

Quantitative analysis of microbleeds using QSM sheds light on the pathophysiological response to the evolution of microbleeds in TBI. One group used QSM analysis of microbleeds in a longitudinal study of 603 military service members with TBI over 0 to 3 months, 3 to 6 months, 6 to 12 months, and greater than 1 year.[37] QSM measures of microbleeds decreased over time: -0.85 mm^3 for total volume and 20 parts per billion per day for mean magnetic susceptibility.[37] This is the first in vivo study to support an innate mechanism to clear the microbleed hemosiderin deposition in patients with TBI. From prior TBI studies using nonquantitative SWI, we learned that there is a propensity for microbleeds to occur peripherally at the gray–white matter junction (Fig. 9). A QSM study using a segmentation approach of the cerebral veins on SWI images showed severe TBI patients have significantly higher segmented venous volumes compared

Artificial Intelligence and Measurement of Microbleed Burden

The depiction, location, and quantification of cerebral microbleeds (CMBs) are important for prognostication and treatment of a myriad of diseases and conditions such as TBI, dementia, and stroke. SWI is a highly sensitive method as it uses the phase information as part of the image contrast. Objects with high susceptibility (like microbleeds) alter the local magnetic field and the phase of local tissue. However, the post-processed image cannot discriminate between a diamagnetic and a paramagnetic source of signal. Using phase maps and QSM in tandem with SWI can aid in CMB detection sensitivity by reducing false positive mimics such as calcium. Using a combination of multiple images, post-processed images, and maps, and even their max/min intensity projections can be time-consuming and prone to errors from human interpretation. Therefore, automated methods are helpful in facilitating both rapid and accurate lesion detection.

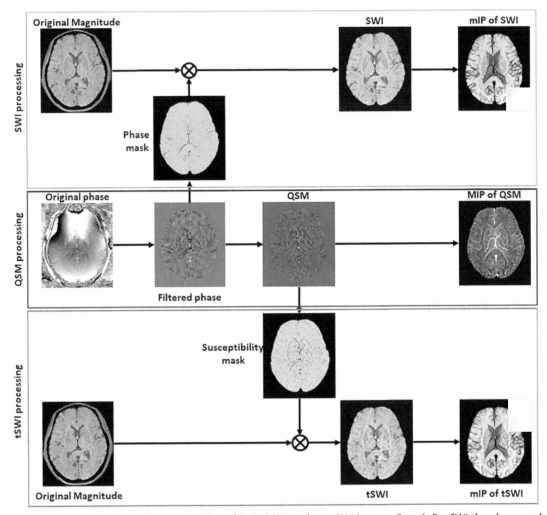

Fig. 7. Flowchart illustrating the construction of SWI, QSM, and true SWI images. Row 1: For SWI the phase mask is multiplied into the original magnitude image four times to produce the SWI data. This can then be mIP over 4 slices were made to better show the continuity of the veins. Row 2: To produce the final QSM data, the phase is first unwrapped and then an inverse process is performed to create the data. These data can then be MIP (maximum intensity projection) over 4 slices were made to again show the veins better. Row 3: The true SWI data are created using a mask from the QSM data rather than from the phase data. This method is able to show the veins at any angle unlike SWI, which cannot highlight the veins at the magic angle of 54.7°. (*Courtesy of* S Buch, PhD, Detroit, MI.)

Liu and colleagues[39] used a two-stage method to detect CMBs on SWI images which involved candidate detection and false positive reduction steps. Their method tested a combination of magnitude, phase, SWI, as well as QSM data as inputs for a convolutional neural network (CNN)-based deep learning technique. The SWI plus phase data performed the best and yielded a high sensitivity (95.8%), a precision of 70.9%, and 1.6 false positives per case which rivals the metrics of human raters and has one of the lowest false positive rates compared with contemporary studies.[39]

The first stage in candidate detection used the SWI images as input and a 3D fast radial symmetry (3D-FRST) method to assess the 'sphericity' of a bleed candidate to help keep punctate-shaped objects and exclude linear objects that may include veins. This involved calculating the fractional anisotropy of the candidate structure in question, and candidates with low FA (close to zero) were chosen for the next stage. The second stage was to reduce false positives in the CNN deep learning model. The SWI plus phase data were fed into the CNN as 32 × 32 x 32 blocks of data. Through a series of convolution functions,

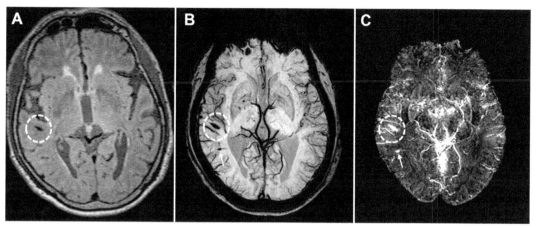

Fig. 8. Patient with TBI demonstrating linear juxtacortical microbleed in the right superior temporal gyrus (*circles*). FLAIR (*A*), mIP SWI (*B*) and Maximum intensity projection (MIP) QSM (*C*) more than eight slices showed increased conspicuity of the microbleed on SWI and QSM. In addition, the SWI and QSM the images found an additional linear microbleed in an adjacent medullary vein which is not visible on the FLAIR (*arrow*). This has been referred to as the "tadpole sign" with the bleed appearing at the end of the vessel.

global and average pooling functions, the data output is either a CMB or a false positive. Each convolution unit was composed of a batch-normalization layer, a Rectified Linear Unit (ReLU), and a 3 × 3 x 3 convolutional layer. For training and validation steps, human raters were considered the gold standard, and 154, 25, and 41 data sets were used for training, validation, and testing, respectively.

This study highlights the importance and value of both deep learning–based methods and using phase information to automate the detection of CMBs with high sensitivity. Clinically, lesion number and load, location, and iron content all have high diagnostic value and can be applied to the aforementioned diseases and conditions. This particular model continues to be trained and optimized using additional inputs such as R2* mapping. The advantage of Liu's study is that data acquired with different sequence parameters with a large variation in CMB size can be used to continue to learn to better detect CMBs and continue reducing false positives (Fig. 10).[39] Many AI and deep learning studies have the disadvantages of either using small data sets or using data from one sequence. Thus, even a deep learning model with a good test performance

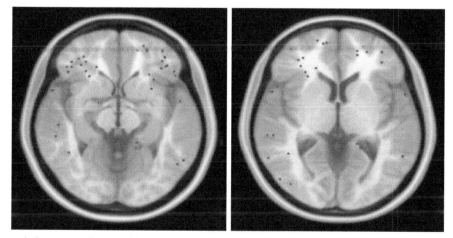

Fig. 9. Example heat maps for 14 mild TBI subjects from a pediatric cohort, which depicts the locations and likelihood of a cerebral microbleeds (CMBs) in the T1 (Montréal neurologic Institute) MNI template space. The CMBs tend to reside in the frontal lobe and to a large degree at the grey-white matter junctions. (Data courtesy of Karen Tong, MD. Loma Linda University.)

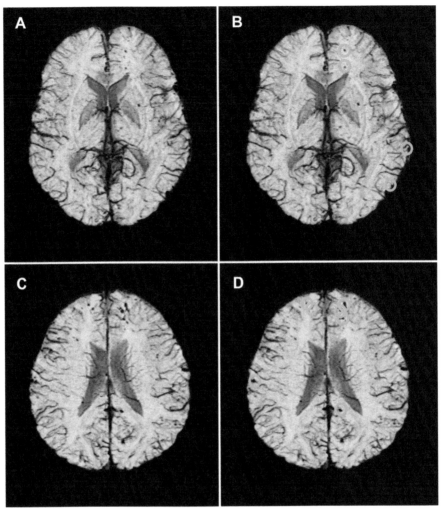

Fig. 10. Results from the microbleed reporting tool from SpinTech's AI algorithm. (*A*, *C*) SWI mIP. (*B*, *D*) overlays of the detected cerebral microbleeds onto (*A*, *C*) represented by green circles.

may not translate to other collected data types from other MR systems or field strengths.

SUMMARY

Several MR imaging techniques have the potential to detect structural and microstructural abnormalities in TBI such as SWI, diffusion tensor imaging, and MR spectroscopy. Each of these modalities along with SWI provides another piece of the puzzle to the complex interaction of the biophysical mechanisms of head injury. SWI and QSM perform the best in the detection of microbleeds, which is the "tip of the iceberg" biomarker of microvascular injuries. QSM and AI offer the ability to detect and follow the evolution of microbleeds in chronic TBI patients, which offers a unique insight into the acute and chronic state of TBI.

DISCLOSURE

The authors have nothing to disclose.

REFERENCES

1. Kirov II, Whitlow CT, Zamora C. Susceptibility-Weighted Imaging and Magnetic Resonance Spectroscopy in Concussion. Neuroimaging Clin N Am 2018;28(1):91–105.
2. Kornguth S, Rutledge N, Perlaza G, et al. A Proposed Mechanism for Development of CTE Following Concussive Events: Head Impact, Water Hammer Injury, Neurofilament Release, and Autoimmune Processes. Brain Sci 2017;7(12):164.
3. Portanova A, Hakakian N, Mikulis DJ, et al. Intracranial vasa vasorum: insights and implications for imaging. Radiology 2013;267(3):667–79.

4. Edwards G 3rd, Zhao J, Dash PK, et al. Traumatic Brain Injury Induces Tau Aggregation and Spreading. J Neurotrauma 2020;37(1):80–92.

5. Edwards G 3rd, Moreno-Gonzalez I, Soto C. Amyloid-beta and tau pathology following repetitive mild traumatic brain injury. Biochem Biophys Res Commun 2017;483(4):1137–42.

6. Haacke EM, Liu S, Buch S, et al. Quantitative susceptibility mapping: current status and future directions. Magn Reson Imaging 2015;33(1):1–25.

7. Haller S, Haacke EM, Thurnher MM, et al. Susceptibility-weighted Imaging: Technical Essentials and Clinical Neurologic Applications. Radiology 2021; 299(1):3–26.

8. Liu S, Buch S, Chen Y, et al. Susceptibility-weighted imaging: current status and future directions. NMR Biomed 2017;30(4):10.

9. Weng CL, Jeng Y, Li YT, et al. Black Dipole or White Dipole: Using Susceptibility Phase Imaging to Differentiate Cerebral Microbleeds from Intracranial Calcifications. AJNR Am J Neuroradiol 2020;41(8): 1405–13.

10. Salmela MB, Krishna SH, Martin DJ, et al. All that bleeds is not black: susceptibility weighted imaging of intracranial hemorrhage and the effect of T1 signal. Clin Imaging 2017;41:69–72.

11. Hsu CC, Haacke EM, Heyn CC, et al. The T1 shine through effect on susceptibility weighted imaging: an under recognized phenomenon. Neuroradiology 2018;60(3):235–7.

12. Conklin J, Longo MGF, Cauley SF, et al. Validation of Highly Accelerated Wave-CAIPI SWI Compared with Conventional SWI and T2*-Weighted Gradient Recalled-Echo for Routine Clinical Brain MRI at 3T. AJNR Am J Neuroradiol 2019;40(12):2073–80.

13. Greenberg SM, Vernooij MW, Cordonnier C, et al. Cerebral microbleeds: a guide to detection and interpretation. Lancet Neurol 2009;8(2):165–74.

14. Vernooij MW, Ikram MA, Wielopolski PA, et al. Cerebral microbleeds: accelerated 3D T2*-weighted GRE MR imaging versus conventional 2D T2*-weighted GRE MR imaging for detection. Radiology 2008;248(1):272–7.

15. Beauchamp MH, Ditchfield M, Babl FE, et al. Detecting traumatic brain lesions in children: CT versus MRI versus susceptibility weighted imaging (SWI). J Neurotrauma 2011;28(6):915–27.

16. Liu G, Ghimire P, Pang H, et al. Improved sensitivity of 3.0 Tesla susceptibility-weighted imaging in detecting traumatic bleeds and its use in predicting outcomes in patients with mild traumatic brain injury. Acta Radiol 2015;56(10):1256–63.

17. Ashwal S, Babikian T, Gardner-Nichols J, et al. Susceptibility-weighted imaging and proton magnetic resonance spectroscopy in assessment of outcome after pediatric traumatic brain injury. Arch Phys Med Rehabil 2006;87(12 Suppl 2):S50–8.

18. Huang YL, Kuo YS, Tseng YC, et al. Susceptibility-weighted MRI in mild traumatic brain injury. Neurology 2015;84(6):580–5.

19. Griffin AD, Turtzo LC, Parikh GY, et al. Traumatic microbleeds suggest vascular injury and predict disability in traumatic brain injury. Brain 2019;142(11):3550–64.

20. Tao JJ, Zhang WJ, Wang D, et al. Susceptibility weighted imaging in the evaluation of hemorrhagic diffuse axonal injury. Neural Regen Res 2015; 10(11):1879–81.

21. Beauchamp MH, Beare R, Ditchfield M, et al. Susceptibility weighted imaging and its relationship to outcome after pediatric traumatic brain injury. Cortex 2013;49(2):591–8.

22. Tong KA, Ashwal S, Holshouser BA, et al. Diffuse axonal injury in children: clinical correlation with hemorrhagic lesions. Ann Neurol 2004;56(1):36–50.

23. Lotan E, Morley C, Newman J, et al. Prevalence of Cerebral Microhemorrhage following Chronic Blast-Related Mild Traumatic Brain Injury in Military Service Members Using Susceptibility-Weighted MRI. AJNR Am J Neuroradiol 2018;39(7):1222–5.

24. Trifan G, Gattu R, Haacke EM, et al. MR imaging findings in mild traumatic brain injury with persistent neurological impairment. Magn Reson Imaging 2017;37:243–51.

25. Park JH, Park SW, Kang SH, et al. Detection of traumatic cerebral microbleeds by susceptibility-weighted image of MRI. J Korean Neurosurg Soc 2009;46(4):365–9.

26. Wang X, Wei XE, Li MH, et al. Microbleeds on susceptibility-weighted MRI in depressive and non-depressive patients after mild traumatic brain injury. Neurol Sci 2014;35(10):1533–9.

27. Panwar J, Hsu CC, Tator CH, et al. Magnetic Resonance Imaging Criteria for Post-Concussion Syndrome: A Study of 127 Post-Concussion Syndrome Patients. J Neurotrauma 2020;37(10):1190–6.

28. Jarrett M, Tam R, Hernandez-Torres E, et al. A Prospective Pilot Investigation of Brain Volume, White Matter Hyperintensities, and Hemorrhagic Lesions after Mild Traumatic Brain Injury. Front Neurol 2016;7:11.

29. Maugans TA, Farley C, Altaye M, et al. Pediatric sports-related concussion produces cerebral blood flow alterations. Pediatrics 2012;129(1):28–37.

30. Ellis MJ, Leiter J, Hall T, et al. Neuroimaging findings in pediatric sports-related concussion. J Neurosurg Pediatr 2015;16(3):241–7.

31. Lee YJ, Lee S, Jang J, et al. Findings Regarding an Intracranial Hemorrhage on the Phase Image of a Susceptibility-Weighted Image (SWI), According to the Stage, Location, and Size. Investigative Magnetic Resonance Imaging 2015;12(2):107–13.

32. Verma RK, Kottke R, Andereggen L, et al. Detecting subarachnoid hemorrhage: comparison of combined FLAIR/SWI versus CT. Eur J Radiol 2013; 82(9):1539–45.

33. Wu Z, Li S, Lei J, et al. Evaluation of traumatic sub-arachnoid hemorrhage using susceptibility-weighted imaging. AJNR Am J Neuroradiol 2010;31(7):1302–10.

34. Gharabaghi S, Liu S, Wang Y, et al. Multi-Echo Quantitative Susceptibility Mapping for Strategically Acquired Gradient Echo (STAGE) Imaging. Front Neurosci 2020;14:581474.

35. Ruetten PPR, Gillard JH, Graves MJ. Introduction to Quantitative Susceptibility Mapping and Susceptibility Weighted Imaging. Br J Radiol 2019;92(1101):20181016.

36. Wang Y, Liu T. Quantitative susceptibility mapping (QSM): Decoding MRI data for a tissue magnetic biomarker. Magn Reson Med 2015;73(1):82–101.

37. Liu W, Soderlund K, Senseney JS, et al. Imaging Cerebral Microhemorrhages in Military Service Members with Chronic Traumatic Brain Injury. Radiology 2016;278(2):536–45.

38. Liu W, Yeh PH, Nathan DE, et al. Assessment of Brain Venous Structure in Military Traumatic Brain Injury Patients using Susceptibility Weighted Imaging and Quantitative Susceptibility Mapping. J Neurotrauma 2019;36(14):2213–21.

39. Liu S, Utriainen D, Chai C, et al. Cerebral microbleed detection using Susceptibility Weighted Imaging and deep learning. Neuroimage 2019;198:271–82.

Imaging of Abusive Head Trauma in Children

Asthik Biswas, MBBS, DNB[a,b,c,]*, Pradeep Krishnan, MBBS, MD[a,b], Ibrahem Albalkhi[c,d], Kshitij Mankad, MBBS, FRCR[c,e], Manohar Shroff, MD, FRCPC, DABR, DMRD[a,b]

KEYWORDS

• Abusive head trauma • MR imaging • Neuroimaging

KEY POINTS

• Abusive head trauma is not a radiological diagnosis and is made following assessment by a multidisciplinary team comprising various specialties such as physicians, surgeons, radiologists, social workers, and child protection services.
• The radiologist often plays the role of "sentinel" expert in raising the possibility of abusive head trauma (AHT), and shares the burden of medical responsibility along with the multidisciplinary team.
• A thorough understanding of the underlying biomechanisms of AHT is necessary to accurately characterize the imaging findings in context.

INTRODUCTION

Abusive head trauma (AHT) is defined by the US Centers for Disease Control and Prevention *as* "an injury to the skull or intracranial contents of an infant or child younger than 5 years caused by inflicted blunt impact, violent shaking, or both".[1] AHT is the foremost cause of mortality in non-accidental injury,[2] with a fatality rate of greater than 20%.[3,4] The incidence rate of AHT from various population studies is estimated to range from 14 to 53 per 100,000 live births.[5]

Although neuroimaging plays a critical role in the diagnosis of AHT, imaging findings must be interpreted by taking into context the history, clinical findings, and relevant laboratory testing. Indeed, a multidisciplinary team (MDT) comprising experts in Emergency Medicine, Pediatrics, Surgery, Orthopedics, Radiology, Child Protection Services, and Forensic Pathology, to name a few, are involved in making the overall diagnosis. The radiologist often plays the role of "sentinel" expert in raising the possibility of AHT, and shares the burden of

medical responsibility along with the MDT. Therefore, a thorough understanding of the underlying biomechanisms and their imaging correlates is necessary to provide the best possible care to patients and their families. In this review, we will discuss briefly imaging modalities for the evaluation of AHT, mechanisms of injury, imaging appearances of AHT, and its mimics.

IMAGING MODALITIES

Imaging of the head for the investigation of AHT is generally performed in the following scenarios: (a) in the setting of history of fall, scalp swelling, or unexplained bruising, unenhanced computed tomography (CT) of the head is often used as the initial screening examination, (b) In cases where the history is unclear, or if the presenting symptom is non-specific such as inconsolable crying, lethargy or encephalopathy; or presentation as a sudden catastrophic event such as apnea and seizures, the initial examination is either CT or MR imaging taking into account the urgency, scanner availability,

[a] Department of Diagnostic Imaging, The Hospital for Sick Children, 555 University Avenue, Toronto, ON M5G 1X8, Canada; [b] Department of Medical Imaging, University of Toronto, Ontario, Canada; [c] Department of Neuroradiology, Great Ormond Street Hospital for Children NHS Foundation Trust, Great Ormond Street, London WC1N3JH, UK; [d] College of Medicine, Alfaisal University, Al Takhassousi Al Zahrawi Street interconnecting with, Riyadh 11533, Saudi Arabia; [e] UCL GOS Institute of Child Health
* Corresponding author. Department of Neuroradiology, Great Ormond Street Hospital for Children NHS Foundation Trust, Great Ormond Street, London WC1N3JH, UK
E-mail address: asthikbiswas@gmail.com

Neuroimag Clin N Am 33 (2023) 357–373
https://doi.org/10.1016/j.nic.2023.01.010

age of the child, and local institutional protocols; and (c) screening of the CNS in children with extracranial injuries suspicious of abuse.

Typically, both CT and MR imaging are performed in the above scenarios, as each technique offers unique advantages over the other to answer specific questions. CT utilizing multiplanar reformatting and volume rendering is exquisitely sensitive in detecting skull fractures. Three-dimensional (3D) CT is now the expected standard of care for detecting fractures, and for delineating normal variants from fractures. CT is also useful in excluding parenchymal hemorrhage, mass effect, midline shift, and herniation. MR imaging is more sensitive than CT for intracranial hemorrhage and fluid collections, focal and diffuse parenchymal injuries, intraspinal injuries, vertebral body trauma, and paraspinal soft tissue injuries.

The imaging protocol for suspected AHT recommended by the Royal College of Radiologists[6] is shown in Box 1. This is the basic protocol that is recommended to be performed in suspected AHT, with addition of sequences as deemed necessary on a case-by-case basis.

Box 1
RCR recommended basic imaging protocol for suspected AHT

Recommended CT protocol

- Unenhanced CT from skull base to vertex utilizing a multi-slice technique
- Multiplanar reconstructions in the true coronal and true sagittal planes must be performed
- 3D surface reconstructions in bone and soft tissue windows should be done for optimal assessment of skull fractures and associated scalp injuries

Recommended MR imaging protocol

Brain

- Sagittal and axial T1
- Axial diffusion-weighted imaging (DWI)
- Axial T2
- Axial or coronal fluid-attenuated inversion recovery (FLAIR)
- Axial T2 gradient echo or susceptibility weighted imaging (SWI)

Spine

- Sagittal T1
- Sagittal T2
- Sagittal short tau inversion recovery (STIR)
- Axial T1 and T2 (as required)

MECHANISMS OF INJURY AND UNIQUE CHARACTERISTICS OF THE INFANT'S HEAD

The biomechanics of trauma in children are unique when compared with adults. In addition, the response of the pediatric skull, brain and neck to trauma varies non-linearly during the period of early development.[7–9] Similarly, the threshold required for imparting injury as well as the ability of the brain to recover from the injury may be a function of the developmental age of the child.[10,11] It is important to highlight here that given the paucity of age-appropriate human specimens available for research, much of our knowledge on the biomechanics of AHT stems from computational modeling that is driven by data from animal and cadaveric experiments.

Two main mechanisms of injuries are recognized in AHT, namely "impulse loading" and "impact loading" injuries (Fig. 1).[12] Impulse loading refers to forces generated by alternating angular accelerations and decelerations of the cranial vault, such as those following violent shaking, and results in shearing injuries to the brain parenchyma and meninges. Impact loading refers to forces generated by direct impact to the head, resulting in skull fractures, parenchymal contusions, and associated hemorrhage. Examples of impact loading include slamming, throwing, striking with an object, and crush injuries.[13]

Several factors contribute to the increased susceptibility of the infant's head to injury compared with the adult population. A large head relative to the body, large subarachnoid spaces, weak neck musculature, and higher water content of the unmyelinated infant brain[14] contribute to an increased potential for shearing injuries; the thin, immature infant skull predisposes it to impact injury,[14,15] whereas the relatively flat infant skull base increases the risk of rotational injury.[16,17] A large head with weak neck musculature also contributes to cervical spine injuries.[14] Other factors such as ligamentous laxity and immature ossification further predispose the infant's cervical spine and craniovertebral junction to injury.[18,19]

IMAGING FINDINGS
Intracranial Cavity

Subdural hemorrhage
The most common intracranial finding in AHT is subdural hemorrhage (SDH). In a recent prospective study, SDH was present in 89% (41/46) of children with AHT.[20] The likely mechanism for SDH in AHT is impulse loading, with violent shaking leading to bridging vein rupture and hemorrhage in the subdural compartment (Fig. 2).[21] SDH is also

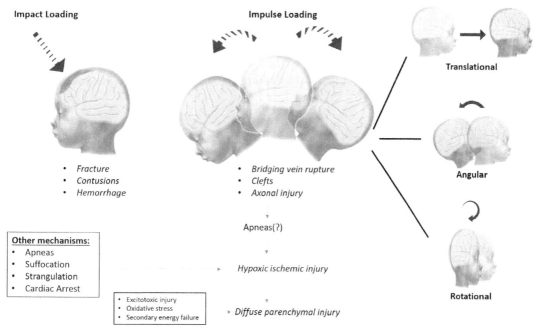

Fig. 1. Mechanisms of injury in abusive head trauma.

frequently seen in accidental head trauma and nontraumatic conditions, and its finding in isolation should therefore be interpreted in the context of other imaging findings. When associated with retinal hemorrhage (RH), hypoxic-ischemic injury (HII), and cerebral edema, the specificity of multiple SDH for AHT increases.[22] Imaging has been shown to identify bridging vein thrombosis in almost half of AHT cases with SDH,[23,24] and the presence of this finding supports a traumatic cause of SDH.[25,26]

SDH in AHT may be unilateral or bilateral, and is often thin, diffuse, and asymmetric, with or without mass effect (Fig. 3). SDH overlying multiple regions, in the interhemispheric region, and posterior fossa have been shown to be significantly associated with AHT.[22] An important region not to be overlooked is the vertex, which is a common site

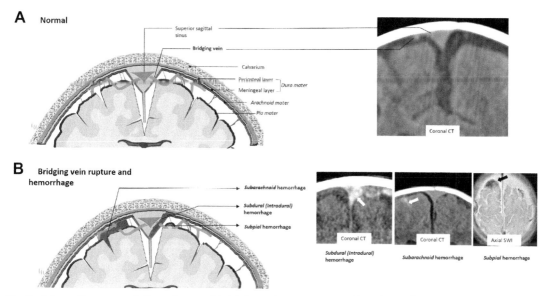

Fig. 2. Schematic representation of normal bridging vein anatomy and its relationship to meningeal layers (A), and bridging vein rupture resulting in different types of hemorrhage (B).

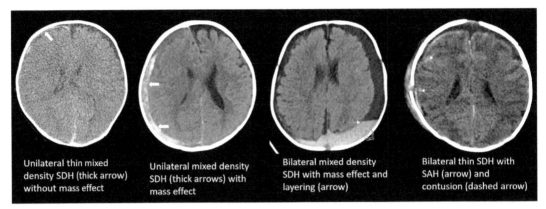

Fig. 3. Patterns of subdural hematoma (SDH) in abusive head trauma.

of bridging vein rupture (Fig. 4) and thrombosis-the imaging features of which are described in the next subsection.

Accurate dating of SDH would be an invaluable evidence in a court of law but unfortunately is fraught with difficulties. There are several reasons for this which include (a) evidence thus far for dating of intracranial hemorrhages on MR imaging is not based on the pediatric population[27]; (b) evolution of extra-axial hemorrhage on MR imaging differs from intraparenchymal hemorrhage; (c) there are broad and overlapping features of SDH at various time points on CT and MR imaging;[28] and (d) acute SDH itself has varying appearances depending on the clotting status (eg, may appear isoattenuating if unclotted), admixture of cerebrospinal fluid (CSF) and blood in case of arachnoid tears (also known as hematohygroma [Fig. 5]),[29–31] and hemoglobin concentration (eg, hypoattenuation in anemia).[32] Indicators of an acute component to the SDH include the presence of hyperdense hemorrhage, rapid change in attenuation, and fluid levels

with the sedimentation of high-density blood products (see Fig. 5A).[33] The absence of these findings however does not necessarily mean the injury is not acute. For instance, a concomitant meningeal tear causes admixture of CSF with blood resulting in hematohygroma and a mixed attenuation of the subdural collection (see Fig. 5). Mixed attenuation SDH can also be seen if there is coexisting acute and hyperacute hemorrhage, acute hemorrhage with sedimentation, and acute on chronic hemorrhage. A description of the attenuation of SDH, and comment on ancillary features such as presence of fluid levels and change in appearance over time is therefore recommended rather than attempting to accurately date each hemorrhage.

Dural border cell layer and the concept of intradural hematoma Although the term SDH is widely accepted in medical literature, evidence from histopathological studies appear to suggest the hemorrhage occurs from splitting of the dural border cell layer, and may therefore be "intradural" rather

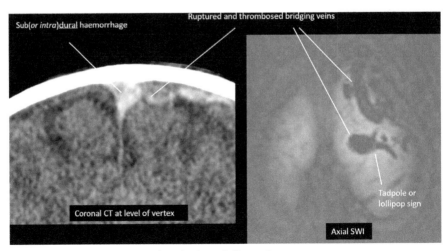

Fig. 4. Bridging vein rupture at vertex with tadpole or lollipop sign.

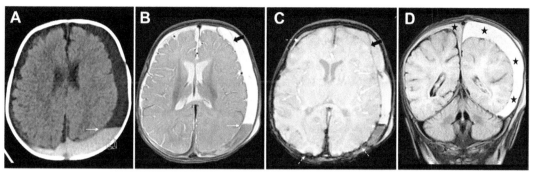

Fig. 5. Hematohygroma. Axial CT image (*A*), T2 (*B*) and susceptibility weighted (*C*) images show mixed density subdural collections bilaterally with a fluid level on the left (*arrows*) with extensive hemosiderin staining (*dashed arrows*, *C*). Note the presence of a membrane (*black arrows*, *B* and *C*). Coronal FLAIR (*D*) image shows its utility in depicting the non-CSF intensity of the subdural collections (*asterisks*, *D*).

than subdural in location (Fig. 6).[34,35] This concept also explains the pathophysiology of membrane development (see Fig. 5B and C) and ongoing blood/fluid extravasation into a chronic "SDH" as follows: inflammatory cells accumulate in response to repair the split dural border cell layer –> results in neomembrane formation –> angiogenic factors promote formation of fragile capillaries within this membrane –> blood leakage as a result of fragile capillaries leads to continued inflammatory response and membrane development –> ongoing exudation of blood and fluid into the membrane lined cavity.[36] Regardless of terminology (ie, subdural versus intradural), the presence of this type of hemorrhage is most likely secondary to a traumatic cause (in the absence of coagulopathy).

Bridging vein rupture and thrombosis-the "tadpole" or "lollipop" sign Rupture of bridging veins results in thrombosis. Imaging can therefore be used to identify discontinuity of the vein.[37,38] Typically, the injured terminal end of the thrombosed vein is larger than the rest of the bridging vein. The round-oval shape of the thrombosed terminal end contiguous with the rest of the enlarged and thrombosed bridging vein has been described as the "tadpole"[24] sign or "lollipop"[23] sign (see Fig. 4). Alternatively, the thrombosed bridging vein may simply appear as an enlarged tubular structure without an enlarged terminal end (see Fig. 4).[24]

Diffuse parenchymal injury
Although isolated diffuse parenchymal injury (DPI) is not specific for AHT (except in cases of

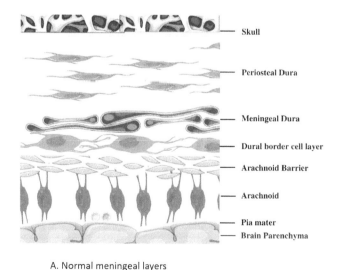

A. Normal meningeal layers

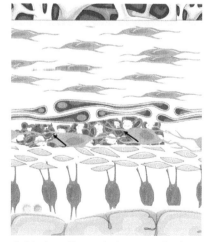

B. Meningeal layers depicting intradural haemorrhage in the <u>dural</u> border cell layer (arrows)

Fig. 6. Schematic diagram showing the normal meningeal layers (*A*), and intradural hemorrhage within the dural border cell layer (*B*).

strangulation or asphyxiation), cerebral edema, hypoxic ischemia, diffuse axonal injury, and closed head injury were found to be statistically significantly associated with AHT as compared with accidental injury.[39] The specificity for AHT increases when DPI is associated with SDH, RH, or cervicomedullary injury.[22,40–43]

Several pathomechanisms have been attributed to DPI in AHT. These include diffuse and focal axonal injury, HII, glutamate-related excitotoxicity, oxidative stress, secondary energy failure, and seizure-mediated injury.[44–47] In reality, the pathophysiology is complex, with several overlapping mechanisms likely contributing to injury (see Figs. 1 and 10).

Diffuse axonal injury is postulated to be caused by rotational and acceleration-deceleration forces, with subsequent failure of axonal transport and excitotoxicity contributing to parenchymal injury.[48] Although DAI was initially considered to be the predominant mechanism of parenchymal injury in AHT, recent studies have revealed that HII occurs more commonly than DAI.[41,45,49,50] Whether focal axonal injury to the respiratory centers of the brainstem and upper cervical cord with subsequent apnea results in, or contributes to HII is unknown but has been postulated as one of the possible pathomechanisms.[51,52] HII can also result from apneas, suffocation, strangulation, and cardiac arrest in the context of AHT.[48]

Excitotoxic injury can result from any process that leads to an increase in extracellular glutamate, such as decreased glutamate reuptake in the settling of energy depletion (HII), increased glutamate release by depolarized neuronal membranes (prolonged seizures), and leakage of glutamate from damaged axons (axonal injury).[53] The immature brain is particularly susceptible to excitotoxic injury given that N-methyl-D-aspartate (NMDA)-type glutamate receptors activity and expression are increased in this age group.[54] Oxidative stress in traumatic brain injury can be precipitated by glutamate-mediated excitotoxicity,[55] tissue disruption, release of nitric oxide synthase (NOS), and dysregulation of electron transport.[56] Secondary energy failure results from excitotoxicity, oxidative stress, and inflammation,[57,58] with the end result being cell death mediated by necrosis, apoptosis, and autophagy.[59]

Imaging findings depend on the nature of the injury and when the imaging is performed following the injury (see Figs. 9–11). Several patterns of HII may be seen such as diffuse cerebral involvement, watershed involvement, and cortical-subcortical patterns,[41,45,49,50] with or without deep gray matter injury (Fig. 7).[49] These can be symmetric or asymmetric (see Fig. 7). Unilateral patterns have also been described and are strongly correlated with AHT in the presence of ipsilateral subdural and RH (Fig. 8).[48,60] The reason for asymmetric and unilateral HII is not completely understood, with transient occlusion or compromise of neck vessels on one side during the event postulated to result in ipsilateral or regional cytotoxic edema.[60] HII may coexist with shearing or impact injuries and vice versa. Indeed, variable appearances are common, and many overlapping features may be present.

Hypoxic injury on an early screening CT may not be readily apparent. Key features to look for are diffuse cerebral edema with effacement of sulci and loss of gray-white matter differentiation (Figs. 9A, B, and 10). Similarly, axonal injury on CT is difficult to diagnose, except in severe cases wherein foci of hyperattenuation may be observed at the gray-white matter junctions, corpus callosum, internal capsule, and brainstem. MR imaging, and in particular diffusion-weighted imaging (DWI), is extremely useful in demonstrating cytotoxic edema of DPI (see Figs. 7, 8A and B, 9C and 10B). Similarly, DWI, susceptibility-weighted imaging (SWI) and gradient recalled echo (GRE) sequences are more sensitive than CT for diagnosing axonal injury (Fig. 11D and E).

Focal parenchymal injury

Focal parenchymal injuries may result from impulse or impact loading mechanisms.[12]

Parenchymal lacerations or clefts occur more commonly in infants younger than 5 months of age, possibly attributable to the increased propensity of the gelatinous white matter for shearing injury at this age.[33,48] They appear as well-marginated CSF and/or hemorrhage-containing cavities in the subcortical white matter or at gray-white matter junctions (see Fig. 9D),[48] generally lined by brain parenchyma all around[61] (compared with clefts from other etiologies). Dependent sedimentation levels may be seen. The frontal lobes are most commonly involved.

Parenchymal contusions result from impact loading. These are less common in infants but can be seen in patients of any age in the setting of direct blunt impact. When present, these are often seen close to the skull base in the frontal and temporal lobes, and adjacent to skull fractures.[12,33] Imaging findings include focal areas of hemorrhage with adjacent edema (see Fig. 11). SWI and GRE sequences are particularly useful for detecting microhemorrhages.

Subarachnoid, subpial, and epidural hemorrhage

Subarachnoid hemorrhage (SAH) in AHT may be due to shearing injury or direct impact. Shearing injury causes tearing of cortical, pial, and arachnoid

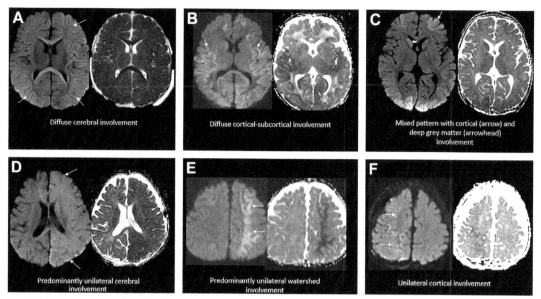

Fig. 7. Patterns of hypoxic ischemic injury in AHT.

vessels and resultant hemorrhage in the subarachnoid space (see Fig. 2). Concomitant tearing of bridging veins along with the arachnoid veins results in the combination of SAH and SDH (see Fig. 3), and are commonly seen along the high cerebral convexities. SAH may also occur secondary to direct impact in which case they are seen adjacent to skull fractures and parenchymal contusions. On imaging, SAH typically hugs the brain and interdigitates into sulci (see Fig. 3) and cisterns. MR imaging with FLAIR, SWI, and GRE sequences are more sensitive than CT for the diagnosis of SAH. Isolated SAH has not been described in AHT.[62,63]

Subpial hemorrhage refers to the accumulation of blood between the pia mater and the cerebral cortex (see Fig. 2). These seem as well-circumscribed areas of bleeding at the edge of a gyrus,[64,65] and in the context of AHT, are seen

adjacent to parenchymal lacerations, SDH and fractures.[12] It can be challenging to differentiate subpial hemorrhage from focal parenchymal contusion and focal SAH on imaging. Generally, subpial hemorrhage overlies cerebral convexity without extension into sulci (see Fig. 2).

Epidural hemorrhage refers to the collection of blood between the inner calvarium and outer periosteal dura. It results from direct impact and is less common when compared with SDH and SAH in the setting of AHT. The mechanism of trauma should therefore be carefully evaluated in the setting of epidural hemorrhage.[66]

Orbits

Retinal hemorrhage
RHs in AHT are postulated to occur from violent shaking, with acceleration and deceleration forces

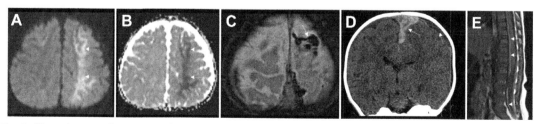

Fig. 8. (Case vignette 1): A 12-month-old boy was brought to the hospital with irritability. History of fall from bed was provided. Axial DWI and ADC images show restricted diffusion involving the left cerebral white matter (arrows, A and B). Axial SWI shows bridging vein rupture and thrombosis (arrow, C) with ipsilateral mixed density subdural hemorrhage (arrows, D). Spinal subdural hemorrhage was also present (arrows, E). Retinal hemorrhage was found on fundoscopy. The case was investigated as suspected AHT on account of discordant imaging findings with the provided history. *Teaching point: Unilateral patterns of HII are strongly correlated with AHT in the presence of ipsilateral subdural and retinal hemorrhage.*

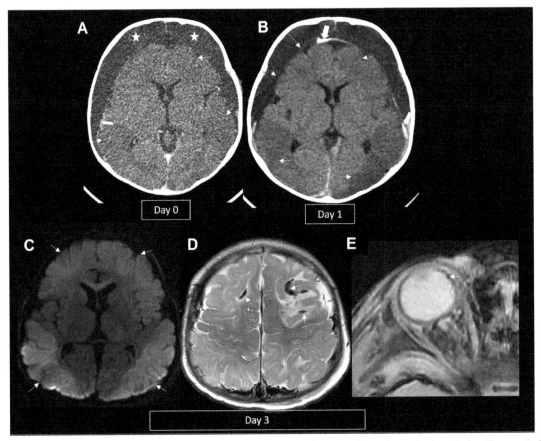

Fig. 9. (Case vignette 2): A 4-month-old lethargic and drowsy infant was brought to the hospital with reported history of having fallen from by approximately 1.5 feet onto a marble floor. Axial CT performed on the day of admission shows subtle loss of gray-white matter differentiation and sulcal effacement (*arrows, A*), bilateral subdural collections (*asterisks, A*) with thin hyperdense blood overlying the surface of the brain (*thick arrow, A*). CT on day 2 of admission shows more clearly the loss of gray-white matter differentiation (*arrows, B*), as well as hyperdense acute blood that was not appreciable on the first CT (*thick arrows, B*) (presumably on account of it being hyperacute blood at that time). CT also shows membranes (*dashed arrows, B*) suggesting the presence of a chronic component to the subdural collections. MR imaging performed on day 4 of admission shows restricted bilateral cerebral restricted diffusion (*arrows, C*), blood filled parenchymal clefts or lacerations at the gray-white matter junctions (*arrows, D*), and retinal hemorrhage (*arrow, E*). Teaching point: This case shows the importance of serial imaging to characterize subdural collections, the utility of diffusion weighted imaging to assess the extent of hypoxic ischemic injury (optimally performed at days 3 to 5 following the presumed hypoxic event), and the higher sensitivity of MR imaging to depict parenchymal lacerations.

resulting in vitreoretinal traction injury.[67,68] RHs that are bilateral, multiple, and multilayered (preretinal, intraretinal, and subretinal), and those that extend peripherally to the ora serrata at fundoscopy are more predictive of an abusive mechanism.[69] Increasing severity of RH is correlated with an increased risk of AHT.[12]

The gold standard for diagnosing RH is a dilated fundoscopic examination. Imaging may provide supportive information to fundoscopy. RHs appear as areas of hyperattenuation on CT and foci of signal drop out on SWI or T2 hypointensity, with or without layering (**Fig. 12**). The sensitivity of MR imaging for detecting RHs is proportional to the

grade of RH, with up to 76% of high-grade RHs detected compared with 14% of low grade-RHs utilizing a standard MR imaging protocol with GRE sequence.[70] Dedicated high-resolution orbital SWI sequence has been shown to have a sensitivity of 83% compared with dilated fundus exam.[71]

Skull Fractures

In both AHT and accidental trauma, linear fractures involving the parietal bone are the most common type of skull fracture (see **Fig. 11**A).[33,72] The presence of this finding alone therefore is not specific to abuse and highlights the

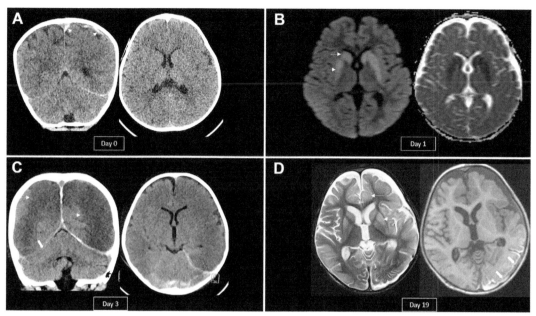

Fig. 10. (Case vignette 3). A 2.5-year-old girl was brought unresponsive to the hospital. The history provided was that she was found face down on the floor following an unwitnessed fall. Coronal and axial CT performed on the day of admission shows subdural hemorrhage along the left vertex (*arrows, A*). No overt loss of gray-white matter differentiation is identified at this time. MR imaging performed one day later shows symmetric restricted diffusion involving the caudate and putamina (*arrows, B*), consistent with profound hypoxic injury. Rest of the cortex appears normal at this time. CT performed on day 3 after admission shows diffuse loss of gray-white matter differentiation with sulcal effacement (*arrows, C*). Note sparing of the cerebellum (*thick arrow, C*). Follow-up MR imaging 19 days following admission shows sequelae of DPI with volume loss, and residual parenchymal T2 hyperintensity (*arrows, D*). Note cortical laminar necrosis (*thick arrows, D*). Teaching point: This case shows the complexity of parenchymal injury in AHT. The initial MR imaging showed hypoxic ischemic injury to the basal ganglia, whereas follow-up imaging showed extensive cortical involvement, suggesting that other factors involved such as secondary energy failure, excitotoxic and oxidative stress induced injury may have contributed to the more delayed DPI in this child. The importance of obtaining follow-up imaging for accurately characterizing the extent of injury is also highlighted in this case, as this has social, medico-legal and prognostic implications.

importance of clinical history and other imaging features. Suspicion of AHT should be raised in the presence of multiple, bilateral, complex, asymmetric diastatic, or depressed fractures in the absence of an appropriate clinical history.[33,72,73]

Imaging criteria used to date long bone fractures cannot be applied to the skull. Also, healing of skull fractures is not significantly accompanied by callus development.[74] In addition, although an adjacent scalp swelling may suggest acuity (see Fig. 11B), the absence of scalp swelling is non-specific and does not predict the timing of skull fracture.[75,76] Using these tools, therefore, at present, it is futile to attempt accurate dating of skull fractures.

Craniocervical Junction and Spine

Spinal injuries have been increasingly recognized in the setting of AHT. As alluded to earlier, several factors such as weak neck musculature and ligamentous laxity contribute to increased propensity for impulse loading type of injuries in the cervical spine. The presence of cervical spine injury in itself cannot aid in distinguishing accidental from non-accidental injury but provides supportive evidence for the traumatic etiology of intracranial SDH.

Ligamentous/soft-tissue injury

The nuchal, interspinous, atlanto-occipital and atlanto-axial ligaments are particularly vulnerable to injury from violent shaking.[40,77] Posterior ligamentous complex damage is more prevalent in AHT when compared with accidental trauma, and suggests that greater forces are involved in the former, possibly representing the result of violent shaking with or without impact.[40,41] Fat-saturated T2-weighted sequences (such as STIR) are useful in demonstrating these injuries (see Fig. 11F).

Spinal subdural hemorrhage

Most spinal SDHs (see Fig. 8E) are thought to occur secondary to gravitation of blood from the intracranial cavity to the most dependent portions of the spine (ie, the thoracolumbar spine).[40] Studies with

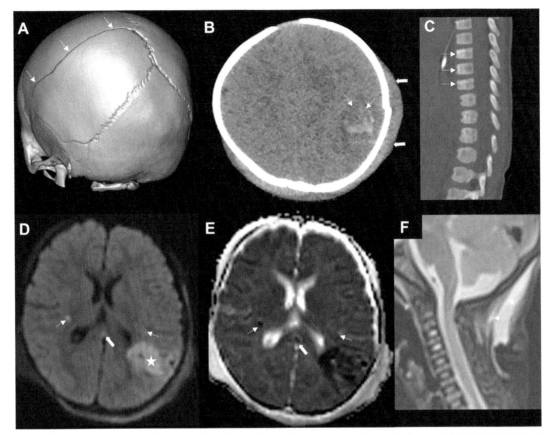

Fig. 11. (Case vignette 4): A 12-month-old girl was brought to the hospital with decreased responsiveness. No clear history of trauma was provided. 3D volume rendered CT image in bone window shows a parietal bone fracture (*arrows, A*). Axial CT image in brain window shows parenchymal hemorrhage (*arrows, B*), and scalp swelling overlying the fracture (*thick arrows, B*). Sagittal CT of the spine in bone window shows multiple lower thoracic compression fractures (*arrows, C*). Axial DWI (*D*) and ADC (*E*) images show punctate foci of restricted diffusion at gray white matter junctions (*arrows, D and E*), and in the splenium of corpus callosum (*thick arrows, D and E*), in addition to the large parenchymal hemorrhage (*asterisk, D*). Sagittal fat saturated T2 weighted image of the cervical spine shows injury to the nuchal ligament (*arrow, F*), with surrounding fluid (*asterisk, F*). Teaching point: This case shows the value of spine imaging in suspected AHT. A fat-saturated T2 or STIR sequence is necessary to diagnose ligamentous injury. A potential pitfall is fluid accumulating in the dependent portion of the suboccipital region as a result of prolonged supine positioning, and care must be taken not to overcall this finding.

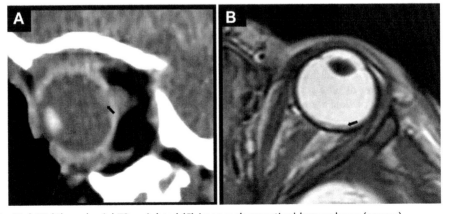

Fig. 12. Sagittal CT (*A*), and axial T2 weighted (*B*) images show retinal hemorrhage (*arrows*).

whole spine imaging[78,79] have shown higher detection rates of spinal SDH compared with studies limited to the cervical spine.[41,80] Furthermore, spinal SDH has been shown to be highly associated with inflicted rather than accidental trauma.[78] It is therefore recommended that imaging for the workup of AHT should include the whole spine.

Spinal fractures

Although uncommon, spinal fractures have been shown with an estimated prevalence of 0.3% to 2.7% in children investigated for suspected child abuse.[81] The prevalence increases to 0.8% to 9.7% in those with a positive skeletal survey.[81] A greater risk of AHT has been calculated in children with spinal fractures than in those without.[82] There appears to be a predilection for vertebral body compression fractures in the thoracic and lumbar spine (see Fig. 11C).[82]

Parenchymal injury

This includes contusions, focal axonal damage, laceration, and nerve root avulsions.[12] The upper cervical spine and brainstem are particularly susceptible to contusions and axonal injury from whiplash-shaking mechanisms.[66] Imaging findings may be subtle and therefore care must be taken to look for these abnormalities, especially when there is associated retroclival hemorrhage, and spinal soft tissue injury.

Retroclival hemorrhage

Retroclival hemorrhage has been shown to occur in about one-third of AHT cases in a large study.[83] Retroclival hemorrhage is commonly associated with injury to the tectorial membrane, and can accumulate anterior (EDH) or posterior (SDH) to the membrane. The presence of retroclival hemorrhage should alert the radiologist to look for other associated craniocervical injuries. Retroclival hemorrhages are best identified on the sagittal plane (Fig. 13).

MIMICS OF ABUSIVE HEAD TRAUMA

A comprehensive review of AHT mimics is beyond the scope of this article. Here we describe some of the common mimics encountered in radiological practice (Fig. 14).

Accidental Injury

Differentiating accidental injury from AHT can be challenging, given that intracranial hemorrhage, parenchymal injury, and skull fractures may be seen in both conditions. In general, SDH from accidental injury tends to be unilateral, adjacent to skull fractures and in association with scalp hematomas, and are considered to result from a

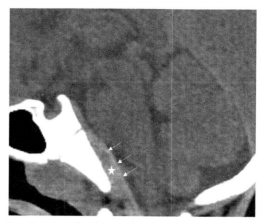

Fig. 13. Retroclival hemorrhage. Sagittal CT shows hyperdense collection (*asterisk*) underlying and lifting the tectorial membrane (*arrows*) away from the clivus.

significant trauma (such as falls from a substantial height).[42] However, short falls with occipital impact have also been shown to result in unilateral SDH.[84] Isolated parietal bone fractures and extradural hemorrhages favor accidental injury over AHT.[22] RHs in accidental trauma tend to be fewer in number, mostly confined to the posterior pole, and are rarely bilateral.[22]

Birth-Related Injury

Clinically silent SDH may arise in term newborns as the result of delivery trauma. These are typically posterior in location, small in size, do not require intervention, generally resolve on imaging by 4 weeks (although residual haemosiderin staining without fluid collection can persist), and have no neurological deficit on follow-up.[85,86] In a study of 88 newborns[87] who had MR imaging following vaginal birth, there was a 26% chance of cerebral bleeding. 16 of the 17 infants who suffered from cerebral bleeding had SDH. In another study,[85] nine (8%) of the 111 newborn infants in a prospective trial who underwent MR imaging within 48 hours of birth had SDH (three vaginal deliveries, five forceps deliveries, and one traumatic vacuum-assisted delivery), none required intervention, and all SDHs resolved at 4-week follow-up MR imaging. The context, clinical history, and outcomes hence help easily differentiate this entity from SDH due to AHT.

Other Conditions Resulting in Subdural Collections

Conditions with enlarged subarachnoid spaces such as benign enlargement of subarachnoid spaces and type 1 glutaric aciduria have the potential to form subdural collections. Similarly,

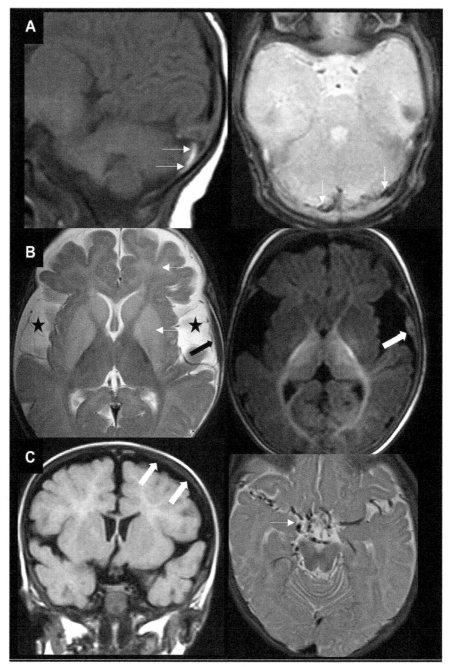

Fig. 14. Mimics of AHT. (A) Thin posterior fossa SDH in a 17 day old neonate (*arrows*). This is commonly seen as a result of birth trauma and resolves spontaneously. (B) Type 1 glutaric aciduria with left temporal SDH (*thick arrows*). SDH occurs due to increased propensity for bridging vein rupture in these patients with enlarged subarachnoid spaces (*asterisks*). Note also basal ganglia and white matter signal abnormality typical of this condition (*arrows*). (C) Subdural collection in Menke's disease (*thick arrows*). Note tortuous arteries of the circle of Willis (*arrows*).

Menke's disease and certain connective tissue disorders can occasionally present with subdural collections mimicking AHT. These mimics are easily differentiated from AHT based on clinical features and other investigations.

Skull Fracture Mimics

Accessory sutures represent normal anatomical variants and occur due to irregular ossification of the calvarium. These are seen most commonly in the parietal and occipital bones on account of an increased number of ossification centers in this region. Sutures appear as nonlinear, interdigitating, serrated lucencies with sclerotic margins, whereas fractures are linear, sharply demarcated lucencies. Other factors that suggest fracture over suture are if the lucency crosses sutures, causes sutural diastasis, or is associated with overlying scalp swelling/hematoma.

Wormian bones are sometimes mistaken for fractures. These represent islands of bone within calvarial sutures and are most commonly related to lambdoid sutures. They are frequently seen as normal variants or may be syndromic, being multiple in number and larger in size in the latter.

CONTROVERSIES

Several theories have been proposed in the recent past to explain the findings seen in AHT. Some of these diagnoses have a scientific basis, and are indeed considered in the differential diagnoses of AHT, such as type 1 glutaric aciduria, Menke's disease, and osteogenesis imperfecta. A careful history, physical examination, MDT approach with appropriate investigations will reliably differentiate these entities from AHT. Other proposed alternative diagnoses such as cerebral venous sinus thrombosis, vitamin D deficiency and Ehlers–Danlos syndrome lack scientific evidence as an explanation of injuries in AHT,[88–90] and therefore remain conjectural hypotheses. Finally, entities such as "temporary brittle bone disease," are completely lacking in evidence and are regarded as purely speculative.[91–93]

CLINICS CARE POINTS 1: PEARLS AND PITFALLS IN INTRACRANIAL IMAGING

- High-resolution coronal susceptibility-weighted imaging is useful in demonstrating traumatic deformation of bridging veins.[37]
- Differentiation of skull fractures from normal variants (sutures and Wormian bones) in the absence of three-dimensional (3D) volume rendered computed tomography (CT) is challenging. Experts agree that 3D CT should be the standard of care.
- Fluid-attenuated inversion recovery imaging, although not routinely performed in infants due to immature myelination, should be added to the MR imaging protocol in suspected abusive head trauma, as it is useful in depicting subdural collections that are not isointense to cerebrospinal fluid.

CLINICS CARE POINTS 2: PEARLS AND PITFALLS IN SPINAL IMAGING

- Fat-saturated T2-weighted or sagittal short tau inversion recovery images should be performed to avoid misdiagnosing normal interspinous fat for fluid.
- Imaging the cervical spine alone may miss spinal subdural hemorrhage as the majority of these are seen in the thoracolumbar region.

CLINICS CARE POINTS 3: OTHER IMPORTANT CONSIDERATIONS

- Abusive head trauma can result in severe brain injury, frequently without a history of serious trauma, and with little to no signs of external injury (e.g. fracture, scalp swelling).[94]
- Following abusive head trauma, hypoxic-ischemic brain injury occurs far more commonly than it does after severe accidental head trauma.[45]
- Injury from a short fall, such from a changing table, bed or sofa, results from translational deceleration and cranial impact.[95] These injuries are typically mild and focal.[84] Serious intracranial injury following these shortfalls is rare, as confirmed by several studies.[96–99]

CLINICS CARE POINTS 4: UNANSWERED QUESTIONS

- The least amount of force necessary to cause the pattern typically linked to abusive head trauma (AHT) is unknown, and experimental attempts to address this issue have clear ethical implications. However, experts largely concur that considerable forces are at play and that minor trauma and routine handling do not contribute to this pattern of severe injury.[100,101] Indeed, repeated use of violent forces has been substantiated by AHT perpetrator confessions.[102]
- The exact mechanism for spinal subdural hemorrhage's is not proven, that is, gravitation to the most dependent portion versus local hemorrhage.

DISCLOSURE

A. Biswas, P. Krishnan, and I. Albalkhi have nothing to disclose. M. Shroff—Occasional medicolegal expert; K. Mankad—offer private medicolegal expertise.

REFERENCES

1. Parks Sharyn E, Annest Joseph L, Hill Holly A, et al. Pediatric abusive head trauma : recommended definitions for public health surveillance and research. National Center for Injury Prevention and Control (US) Division of Violence Prevention; 2012.
2. Keenan Heather T, Runyan Desmond K, Marshall Stephen W, et al. A population-based comparison of clinical and outcome characteristics of young children with serious inflicted and noninflicted traumatic brain injury. Pediatrics 2004;114(3): 633–9.
3. Henry K, Dias Mark S, Shaffer Michele, et al. Demographics of abusive head trauma in the Commonwealth of Pennsylvania. J Neurosurg Pediatr 2008;1(5):351–6.
4. Keenan Heather T, Runyan Desmond K, Marshall Stephen W, et al. A population-based study of inflicted traumatic brain injury in young children. JAMA 2003;290(5):621–6.
5. Biswas A, Shroff Manohar M. Abusive head trauma: Canadian and global perspectives. Pediatr Radiol 2021;51(6):876–82.
6. Royal College of Radiologists and the Society and College of Radiographers, 2017. The radiological investigation of suspected physical abuse in children Available at: https://www.rcr.ac.uk/publication/radiological-investigation-suspected-physical-abusechildren. Accessed October 06, 2022.
7. Brittany C, Margulies Susan S. Material Properties of Human Infant Skull and Suture at High Rates. J Neurotrauma 2006;23(8):1222–32.
8. Luck Jason F, Nightingale Roger W, Loyd Andre M, et al. Tensile mechanical properties of the perinatal and pediatric PMHS osteoligamentous cervical spine. Stapp Car Crash J 2008;52:107–34.
9. McPherson GK, Kriewall TJ. The elastic modulus of fetal cranial bone: a first step towards an understanding of the biomechanics of fetal head molding. J Biomech 1980;13(1):9–16.
10. Ibrahim Nicole G, Jill R, Smith C, et al. Physiological and pathological responses to head rotations in toddler piglets. J Neurotrauma 2010;27(6):1021–35.
11. Symeon M, Harris Brent T, Dodge Carter P, et al. Scaled cortical impact in immature swine: effect of age and gender on lesion volume. J Neurotrauma 2009;26(11):1943–51.
12. Wright Jason N. CNS injuries in abusive head trauma. AJR Am J Roentgenol 2017;208(5):991–1001.
13. Spencer GC. Abusive head trauma: a review of the evidence base. Am J Roentgenol 2015;204(5): 967–73. https://doi.org/10.2214/AJR.14.14191.
14. Susan M, Brittany C. Experimental injury biomechanics of the pediatric head and brain. In: Crandall Jeff R, Myers Barry S, Meaney David F, et al, editors. Pediatric injury biomechanics: archive & textbook. New York, NY: Springer; 2013. p. 157–89.
15. Burgos-Flórez FJ, Garzón-Alvarado DA. Stress and strain propagation on infant skull from impact loads during falls: a finite element analysis. Int Biomech 2020;7(1):19–34.
16. Case Mary E. Distinguishing accidental from inflicted head trauma at autopsy. Pediatr Radiol 2014;44(Suppl 4):S632–40.
17. Case ME, Graham MA, Handy TC, et al. Position paper on fatal abusive head injuries in infants and young children. Am J Forensic Med Pathol 2001;22(2):112–22.
18. Kasai T, Ikata T, Katoh S, et al. Growth of the cervical spine with special reference to its lordosis and mobility. Spine 1996;21(18):2067–73.
19. Bailey Donald K. The Normal Cervical Spine in Infants and Children. Radiology 1952;59(5):712–9.
20. Manuela F, Ulrich L. Shaken baby syndrome in Switzerland: results of a prospective follow-up study, 2002-2007. Eur J Pediatr 2010;169(8):1023–8.
21. Miller Jimmy D, Remi N. Acute subdural hematoma from bridging vein rupture: a potential mechanism for growth: Clinical article. J Neurosurg 2014; 120(6):1378–84.
22. Kemp AM, Jaspan T, Griffiths J, et al. Neuroimaging: what neuroradiological features distinguish abusive from non-abusive head trauma? A systematic review. Arch Dis Child 2011;96(12):1103–12.
23. Choudhary Arabinda K, Ray B, Dias Mark S, et al. Venous injury in abusive head trauma. Pediatr Radiol 2015;45(12):1803–13.
24. Hahnemann Maria L, Sonja K, Bernd S, et al. Imaging of bridging vein thrombosis in infants with abusive head trauma: the "Tadpole Sign. Eur Radiol 2015;25(2):299–305.
25. Caroline R. Bridging veins and autopsy findings in abusive head trauma. Pediatr Radiol 2015;45(8): 1126–31.
26. Catherine A, Caroline R. Abusive head trauma: don't overlook bridging vein thrombosis. Pediatr Radiol 2012;42(11):1298–300.
27. Sieswerda-Hoogendoorn T, Stephen B, Betty S, et al. Abusive head trauma Part II: radiological aspects. Eur J Pediatr 2012;171(4):617–23.
28. Sieswerda-Hoogendoorn T, Postema Floor AM, Dagmar V, et al. Age determination of subdural hematomas with CT and MRI: a systematic review. Eur J Radiol 2014;83(7):1257–68.
29. Joy HM, Anscombe AM, Gawne-Cain ML. Bloodstained, acute subdural hygroma mimicking a

subacute subdural haematoma in non-accidental head injury. Clin Radiol 2007;62(7):703–6.

30. Offiah C, St Clair Forbes W, Thorne J. Non-haemorrhagic subdural collection complicating rupture of a middle cranial fossa arachnoid cyst. Br J Radiol 2006;79(937):79–82.

31. Wittschieber D, Karger B, Niederstadt T, et al. Subdural hygromas in abusive head trauma: pathogenesis, diagnosis, and forensic implications. AJNR Am J Neuroradiol 2015;36(3):432–9.

32. Gilbert V. Assessment of the nature and age of subdural collections in nonaccidental head injury with CT and MRI. Pediatr Radiol 2009;39(6):586–90.

33. Gunda D, Cornwell Benjamin O, Dahmoush Hisham M, et al. Pediatric Central Nervous System Imaging of Nonaccidental Trauma: Beyond Subdural Hematomas. Radiographics 2019;39(1):213–28.

34. Haines DE, Harkey HL, al-Mefty O. The "subdural" space: a new look at an outdated concept. Neurosurgery 1993;32(1):111–20.

35. Tetsumori Y. The Inner Membrane of Chronic Subdural Hematomas: Pathology and Pathophysiology. Neurosurg Clin 2000;11(3):413–24.

36. Ellie E, Giorgi-Coll S, Whitfield Peter C, et al. Pathophysiology of chronic subdural haematoma: inflammation, angiogenesis and implications for pharmacotherapy. J Neuroinflammation 2017; 14(1):108.

37. Giulio Z, Khan Abdullah S, Ashok P, et al. In Vivo Demonstration of Traumatic Rupture of the Bridging Veins in Abusive Head Trauma. Pediatr Neurol 2017;72:31–5.

38. George Koshy V, Sateesh J, Desai S, et al. Venous injury in pediatric abusive head trauma: a pictorial review. Pediatr Radiol 2021;51(6):918–26.

39. Child Protection Evidence Systematic review on Head and Spinal Injuries 2019.

40. Choudhary Arabinda K, Ramsay I, Zacharia Thomas T, et al. Imaging of spinal injury in abusive head trauma: a retrospective study. Pediatr Radiol 2014;44(9):1130–40.

41. Nadja K, Zarir K, Gilbert V, et al. Usefulness of MRI detection of cervical spine and brain injuries in the evaluation of abusive head trauma. Pediatr Radiol 2014;44(7):839–48.

42. Piteau Shalea J, Ward Michelle GK, Barrowman Nick J, et al. Clinical and radiographic characteristics associated with abusive and nonabusive head trauma: a systematic review. Pediatrics 2012; 130(2):315–23.

43. Kelly P, Simon J, Vincent Andrea L, et al. Abusive head trauma and accidental head injury: a 20-year comparative study of referrals to a hospital child protection team. Arch Dis Child 2015; 100(12):1123–30.

44. Ellen GP. Abusive head trauma: parenchymal injury. In: Kleinman Paul K, editor. Diagnostic imaging of child abuse. 3rd edition. Cambridge (United Kingdom): Cambridge University Press; 2015. p. 1165.

45. Ichord Rebecca N, Maryam N, Pollock Avrum N, et al. Hypoxic-ischemic injury complicates inflicted and accidental traumatic brain injury in young children: the role of diffusion-weighted imaging. J Neurotrauma 2007;24(1):106–18.

46. Ruppel Randall A, Clark Robert SB, Hülya Bayir, et al. Critical mechanisms of secondary damage after inflicted head injury in infants and children. Neurosurg Clin N Am 2002;13(2):169–82.

47. Ruppel RA, Kochanek PM, Adelson PD, et al. Excitatory amino acid concentrations in ventricular cerebrospinal fluid after severe traumatic brain injury in infants and children: the role of child abuse. J Pediatr 2001;138(1):18–25.

48. Oates Adam J, Jai S, Kshitij M. Parenchymal brain injuries in abusive head trauma. Pediatr Radiol 2021;51(6):898–910.

49. Emanuele O', Huisman Thierry AGM. Izbudak izlem. prevalence, patterns, and clinical relevance of hypoxic-ischemic injuries in children exposed to abusive head trauma. J Neuroimaging 2018;28(6): 608–14.

50. Zimmerman RA, Bilaniuk LT, Farina L. Non-accidental brain trauma in infants: diffusion imaging, contributions to understanding the injury process. J Neuroradiol 2007;34(2):109–14.

51. Jakob M, Andreas B, Markus B, et al. Encephalopathy and death in infants with abusive head trauma is due to hypoxic-ischemic injury following local brain trauma to vital brainstem centers. Int J Legal Med 2015;129(1):105–14.

52. Adams JH, Doyle D, Ford I, et al. Diffuse axonal injury in head injury: definition, diagnosis and grading. Histopathology 1989;15(1):49–59.

53. Toshio M, Smoker Wendy RK, Sato Yutaka, et al. Diffusion-Weighted Imaging of Acute Excitotoxic Brain Injury. Am J Neuroradiol 2005;26(2):216–28.

54. Waters Karen A, Rita M. NMDA Receptors In the Developing Brain and Effects of Noxious Insults. Nippon Suisan Gakkaish 2004;13(4):162–74.

55. Parfenova H, Shyamali B, Bhattacharya S, et al. Glutamate induces oxidative stress and apoptosis in cerebral vascular endothelial cells: contributions of HO-1 and HO-2 to cytoprotection. Am J Physiol, Cell Physiol 2006;290(5):C1399–410.

56. Hülya B, Kochanek Patrick M, Kagan Valerian E. Oxidative stress in immature brain after traumatic brain injury. Dev Neurosci 2006;28(4–5):420–31.

57. Allen Kimberly A, Brandon Debra H. Hypoxic ischemic encephalopathy: pathophysiology and experimental treatments. Newborn Infant Nurs Rev 2011;11(3):125–33.

58. Perlman JM. Pathogenesis of hypoxic-ischemic brain injury. J Perinatol 2007;27(1):S39–46.

59. Thornton C, Bryan L, Carina M, et al. Cell Death in the Developing Brain after Hypoxia-Ischemia. Front Cell Neurosci 2017;11.

60. McKinney Alexander M, Thompson Linda R, Truwit Charles L, et al. Unilateral hypoxic-ischemic injury in young children from abusive head trauma, lacking craniocervical vascular dissection or cord injury. Pediatr Radiol 2008;38(2):164–74.

61. Jaspan T, Narborough G, Punt JA, et al. Cerebral contusional tears as a marker of child abuse–detection by cranial sonography. Pediatr Radiol 1992;22(4):237–45.

62. Geddes JF, Hackshaw AK, Vowles GH, et al. Neuropathology of inflicted head injury in children. I. Patterns of brain damage. Brain 2001;124(Pt 7):1290–8.

63. Foerster Bradley R, Myria P, Lin D, et al. Neuroimaging evaluation of non-accidental head trauma with correlation to clinical outcomes: a review of 57 cases. J Pediatr 2009;154(4):573–7.

64. Huang Amy H, Robertson Richard L. Spontaneous superficial parenchymal and leptomeningeal hemorrhage in term neonates. AJNR Am J Neuroradiol 2004;25(3):469–75.

65. Cain Donald W, Dingman Andra L, Armstrong Jennifer, et al. Subpial Hemorrhage of the Neonate. Stroke 2020;51(1):315–8.

66. Gunes O, Kralik Stephen F, Avner M, et al. MRI Findings in Pediatric Abusive Head Trauma: A Review. J Neuroimaging 2020;30(1):15–27.

67. Levin Alex V. Retinal hemorrhage in abusive head trauma. Pediatrics 2010;126(5):961–70.

68. Gil B, Forbes Brian J. The eye in child abuse: key points on retinal hemorrhages and abusive head trauma. Pediatr Radiol 2014;44(Suppl 4):S571–7.

69. Maguire SA, Watts PO, Shaw AD, et al. Retinal haemorrhages and related findings in abusive and non-abusive head trauma: a systematic review. Eye 2013;27(1):28–36.

70. Beavers Angela J, Stagner Anna M, Allbery Sandra M, et al. MR detection of retinal hemorrhages: correlation with graded ophthalmologic exam. Pediatr Radiol 2015;45(9):1363–71.

71. Giulio Z, Ashok P, Anshul H, et al. Susceptibility weighted imaging depicts retinal hemorrhages in abusive head trauma. Neuroradiology 2013;55(7):889–93.

72. Kemp Alison M, Frank D, Harrison S, et al. Patterns of skeletal fractures in child abuse: systematic review. BMJ 2008;337:a1518.

73. Hobbs CJ. Skull fracture and the diagnosis of abuse. Arch Dis Child 1984;59(3):246–52.

74. Harper Nancy S, Sonja E, Shukla K, et al. Radiologic assessment of skull fracture healing in young children. Pediatr Emerg Care 2021;37(4):213–7.

75. Metz James B, Otjen Jeffrey P, Perez Francisco A, et al. Fracture-associated bruising and soft tissue swelling in young children with skull fractures: how sensitive are they to fracture presence? Pediatr Emerg Care 2021;37(12):e1392–6.

76. Ibrahim Nicole G, Wood J, Margulies Susan S, et al. Influence of age and fall type on head injuries in infants and toddlers. Int J Dev Neurosci 2012;30(3):201–6.

77. Jacob R, Cox M, Koral K, et al. MR imaging of the cervical spine in nonaccidental trauma: a tertiary institution experience. Am J Neuroradiol 2016;37(10):1944–50.

78. Kumar CA, Bradford Ray K, Dias Mark S, et al. Spinal subdural hemorrhage in abusive head trauma: a retrospective study. Radiology 2012;262(1):216–23.

79. Koumellis P, McConachie NS, Jaspan T. Spinal subdural haematomas in children with non-accidental head injury. Arch Dis Child 2009;94(3):216–9.

80. Feldman KW, Weinberger E, Milstein JM, et al. Cervical spine MRI in abused infants. Child Abuse Negl 1997;21(2):199–205.

81. Kemp A, Laura C, Sabine M. Spinal injuries in abusive head trauma: patterns and recommendations. Pediatr Radiol 2014;44(Suppl 4):S604–12.

82. Barber I, Perez-Rossello Jeannette M, Wilson Celeste R, et al. Prevalence and relevance of pediatric spinal fractures in suspected child abuse. Pediatr Radiol 2013;43(11):1507–15.

83. Michelle SV, Danehy Amy R, Newton Alice W, et al. Retroclival collections associated with abusive head trauma in children. Pediatr Radiol 2014;44(Suppl 4):S621–31.

84. Atkinson N, van Rijn Rick R, Starling Suzanne P. Childhood falls with occipital impacts. Pediatr Emerg Care 2018;34(12):837–41.

85. Whitby EH, Griffiths PD, Rutter S, et al. Frequency and natural history of subdural haemorrhages in babies and relation to obstetric factors. Lancet 2004;363(9412):846–51.

86. Rooks VJ, Eaton JP, Ruess L, et al. Prevalence and evolution of intracranial hemorrhage in asymptomatic term infants. AJNR Am J Neuroradiol 2008;29(6):1082–9.

87. Looney Christopher B, Smith J, Keith, Merck Lisa H, et al. Intracranial hemorrhage in asymptomatic neonates: prevalence on MR images and relationship to obstetric and neonatal risk factors. Radiology 2007;242(2):535–41.

88. McLean LA, Frasier LD, Hedlund GL. Does Intracranial Venous Thrombosis Cause Subdural Hemorrhage in the Pediatric Population? Am J Neuroradiol 2012;33(7):1281–4.

89. Chapman T, Sugar N, Stephen D, et al. Fractures in infants and toddlers with rickets. Pediatr Radiol 2010;40(7):1184–9.

90. Marco C. Ehlers-Danlos syndrome(s) mimicking child abuse: Is there an impact on clinical practice? Am J Med Genet C Semin Med Genet 2015;169(4):289–92.

91. Leventhal John M, Edwards George A. Flawed theories to explain child physical abuse: what are the medical-legal consequences? JAMA 2017;318(14):1317–8.

92. Edwards George A. Mimics of child abuse: Can choking explain abusive head trauma? J Forensic Leg Med 2015;35:33–7.

93. Marcovitch H, Mughal Mz. Cases do not support temporary brittle bone disease. Acta Paediatr 2010;99(4):485–6.

94. Narang Sandeep K, Amanda F, James L, et al. Abusive Head Trauma in Infants and Children. Pediatrics 2020;145(4):e20200203.

95. Ommaya AK, Gennarelli TA. Cerebral concussion and traumatic unconsciousness. Correlation of experimental and clinical observations of blunt head injuries. Brain 1974;97(4):633–54.

96. Nimityongskul P, Anderson LD. The likelihood of injuries when children fall out of bed. J Pediatr Orthop 1987;7(2):184–6.

97. Helfer RE, Slovis TL, Black M. Injuries resulting when small children fall out of bed. Pediatrics 1977;60(4):533–5.

98. Lyons TJ, Oates RK. Falling out of bed: a relatively benign occurrence. Pediatrics 1993;92(1):125–7.

99. Chadwick David L, Gina B, Castillo E, et al. Annual risk of death resulting from short falls among young children: less than 1 in 1 million. Pediatrics 2008;121(6):1213–24.

100. Richards PG, Bertocci GE, Bonshek RE, et al. Shaken baby syndrome. Arch Dis Child 2006;91(3):205–6.

101. Harding B, Anthony RR, Krous Henry F. Shaken baby syndrome. BMJ 2004;328(7442):720–1.

102. Catherine A, Sophie G, Nathalie M, et al. Abusive head trauma: judicial admissions highlight violent and repetitive shaking. Pediatrics 2010;126(3):546–55.

Printed and bound by CPI Group (UK) Ltd, Croydon, CR0 4YY

03/10/2024

01040367-0012